Look at Our Plate

A Balanced Meal!

Story by Monique Dorcely

All rights reserved. No part of this publication may be reproduced or transmitted in any form or by any means, electronic or mechanical, including photocopy, recording, taping, or any information storage and retrieval system, without permission from the publisher.

https://pathtogrowllc.com/

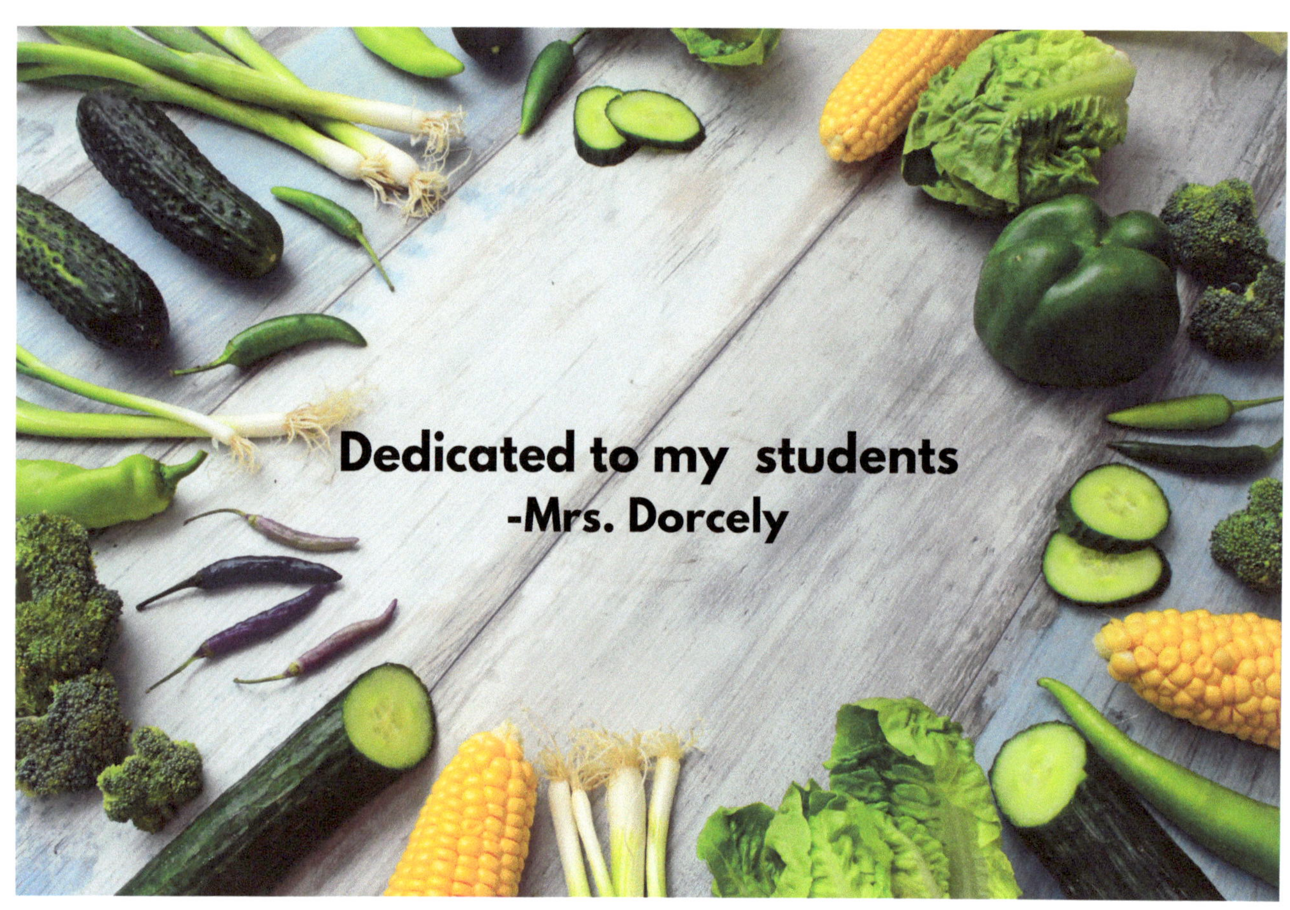
Dedicated to my students
-Mrs. Dorcely

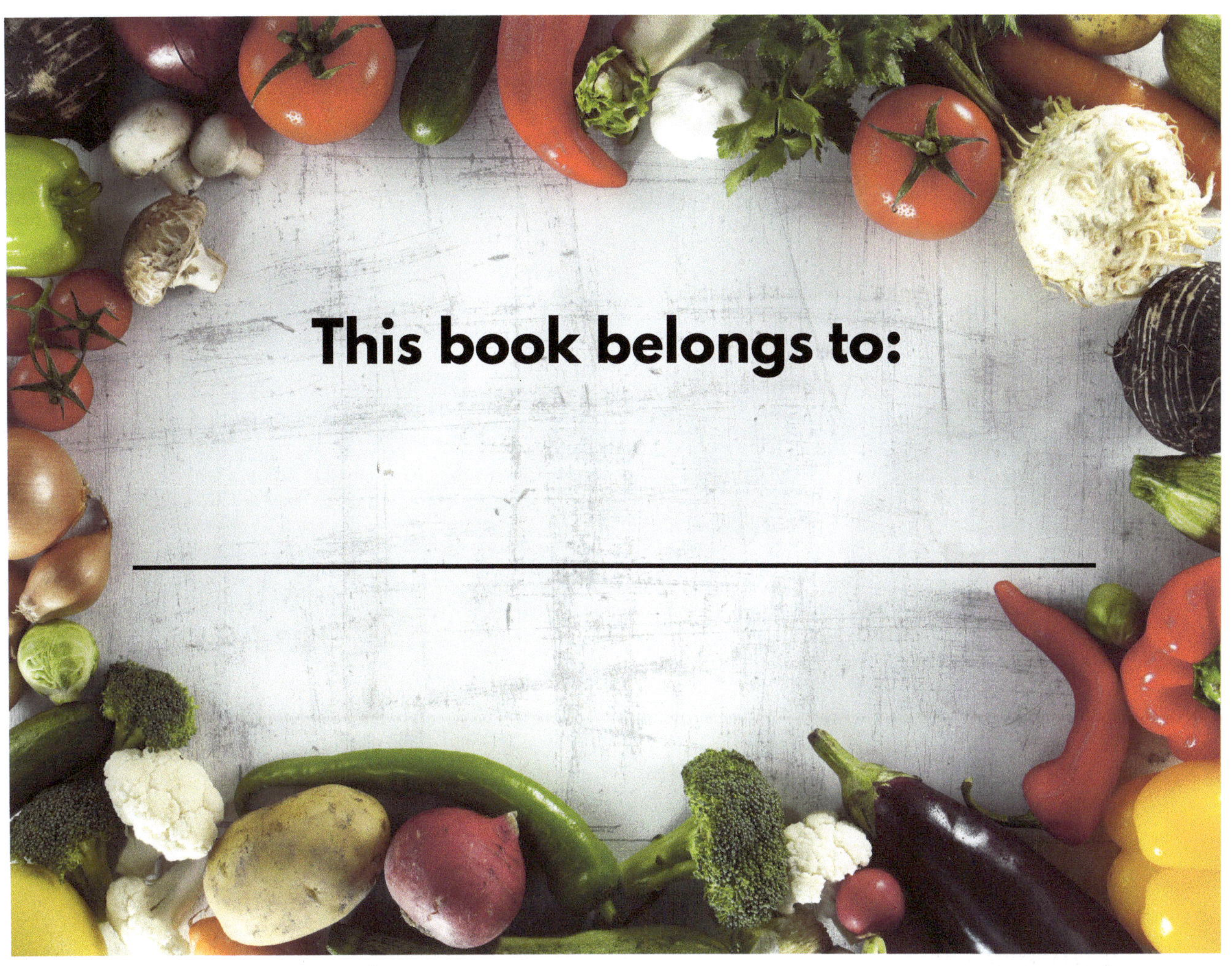
This book belongs to:

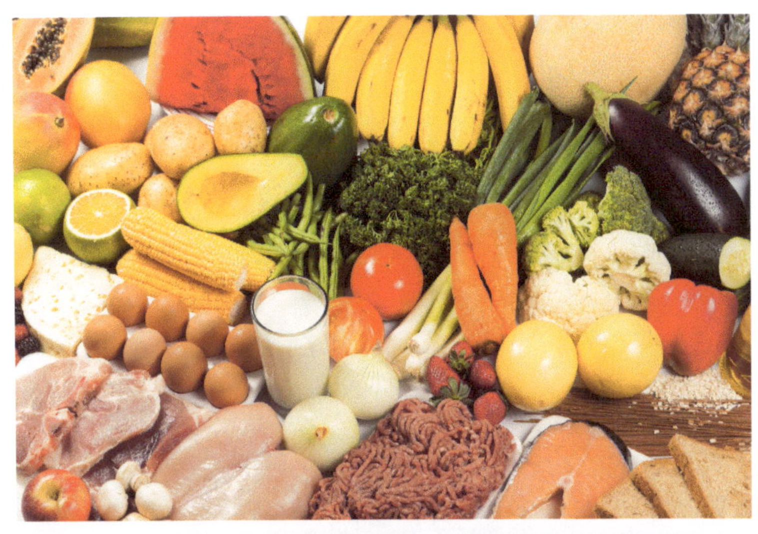

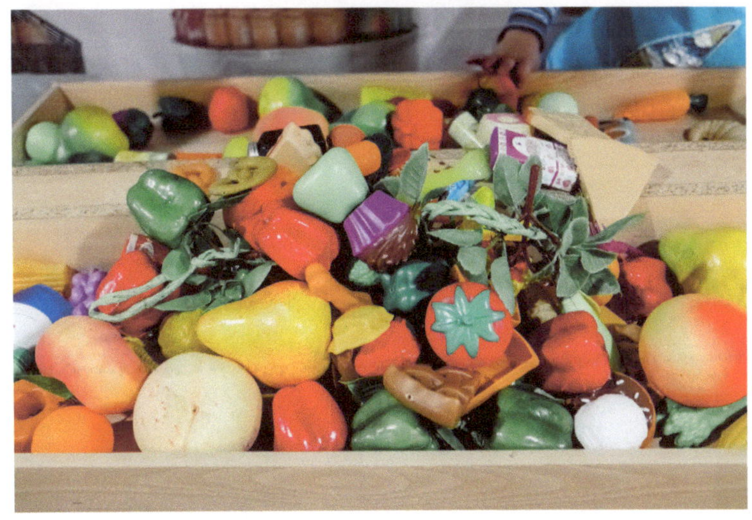

**Ms. D says, “This week is our food fair.
We are learning about the food groups.”
She brings real food and play food to class.**

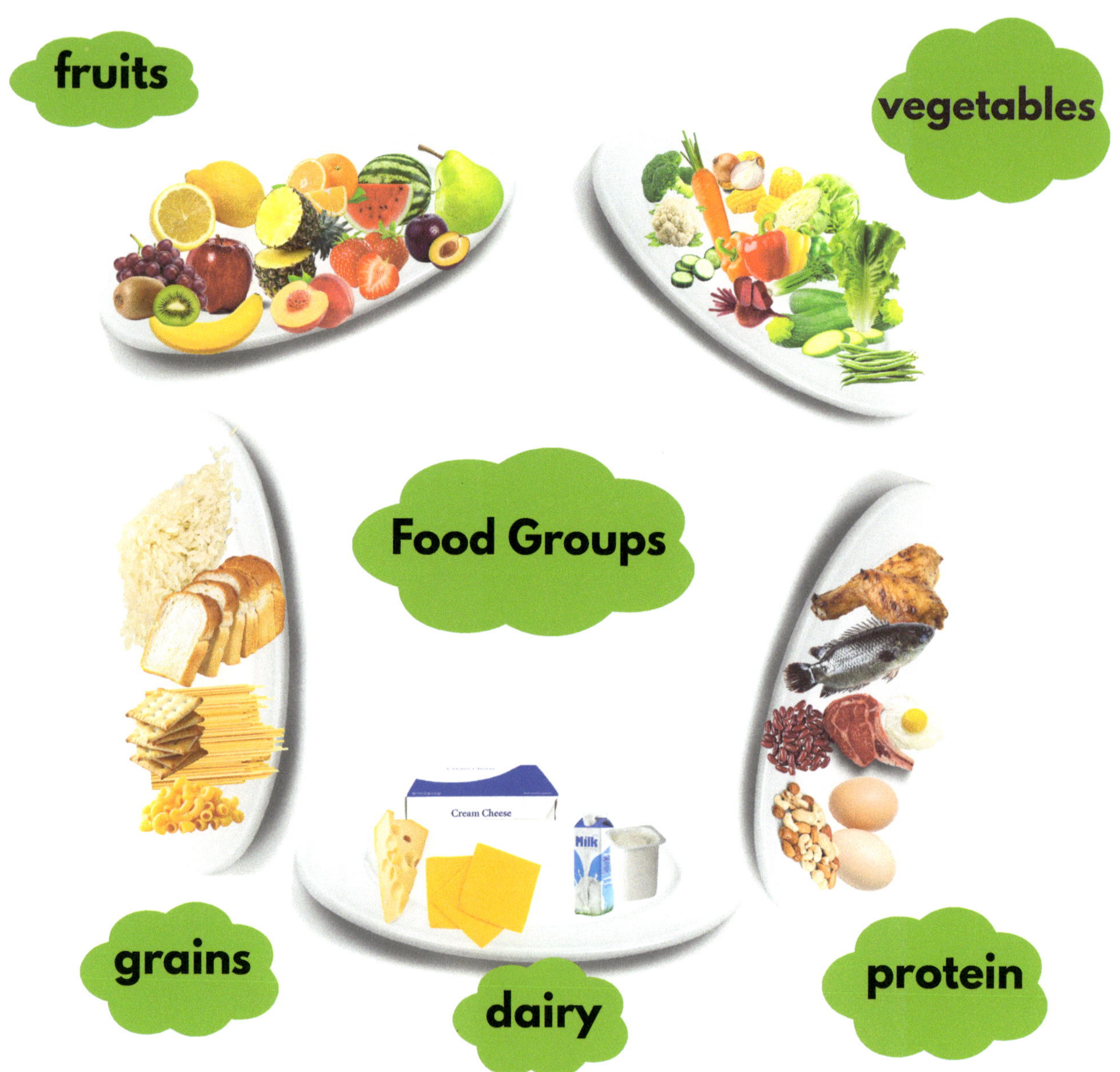

The students sort the food into food groups.

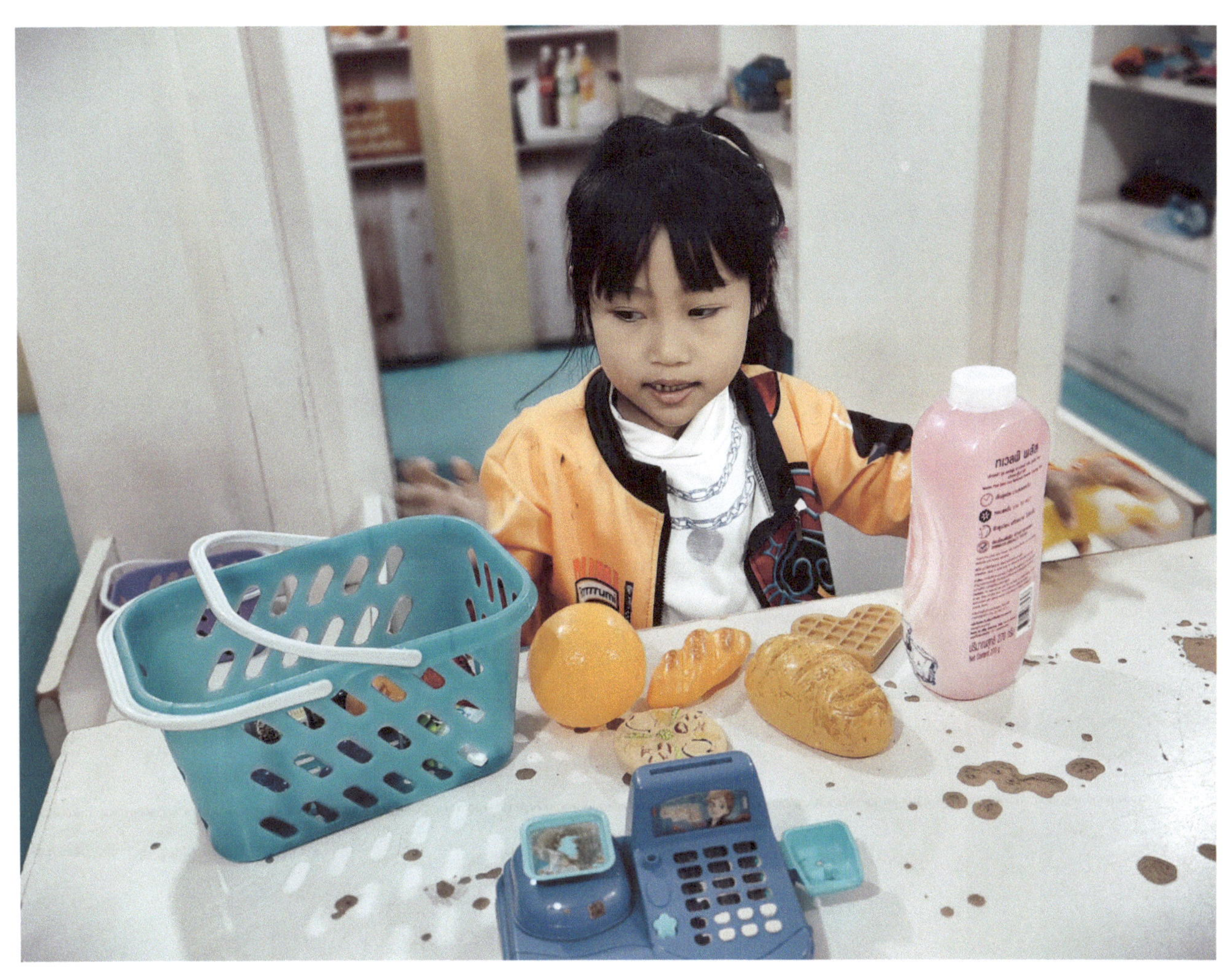

We turn our classroom into a grocery store.

Grocery List

Dairy	Grains	Protein	Vegetables	Fruits
cheese	muffin	eggs	broccoli	orange
milk	pasta	meat	carrot	appple
cream cheese	bread	beans	potato	banana

We make a grocery list.

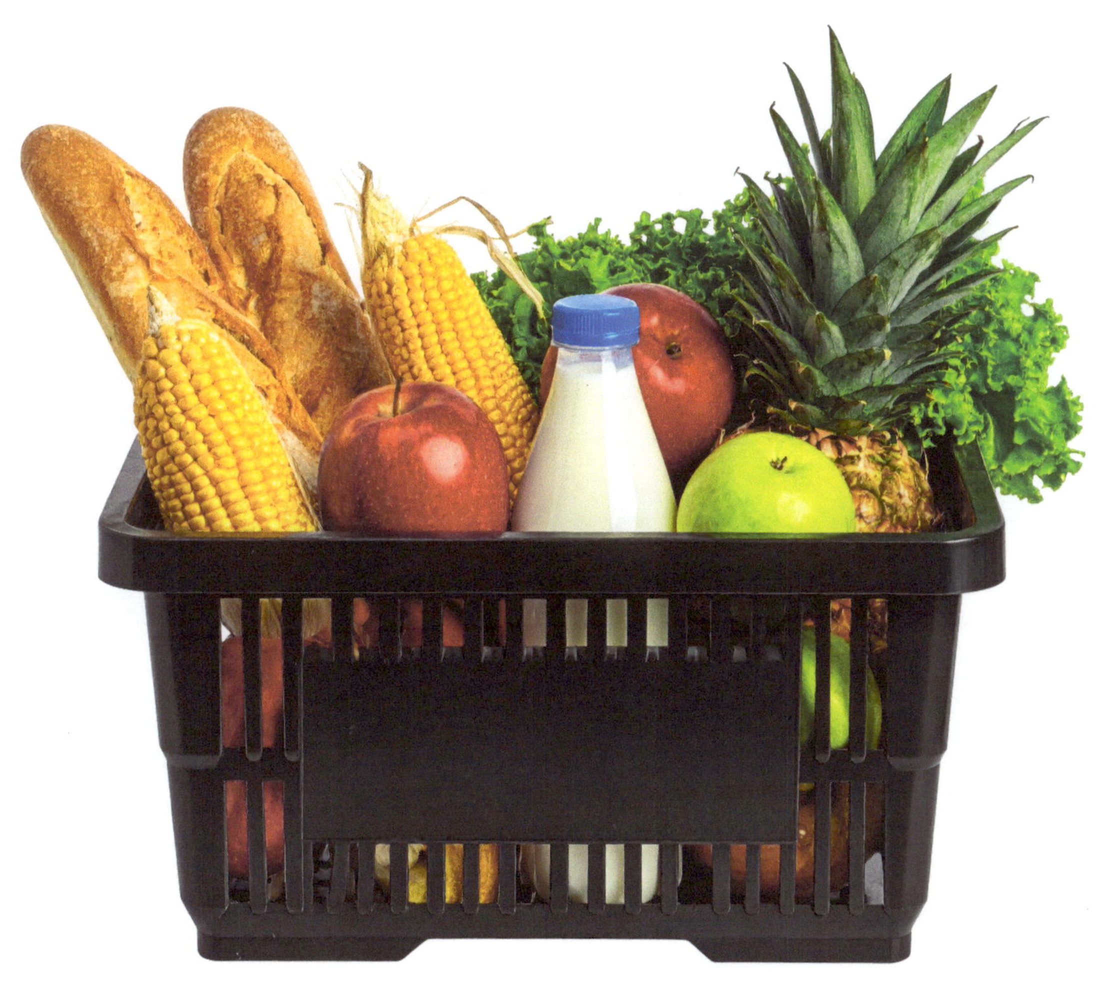

We shop at the grocery store.

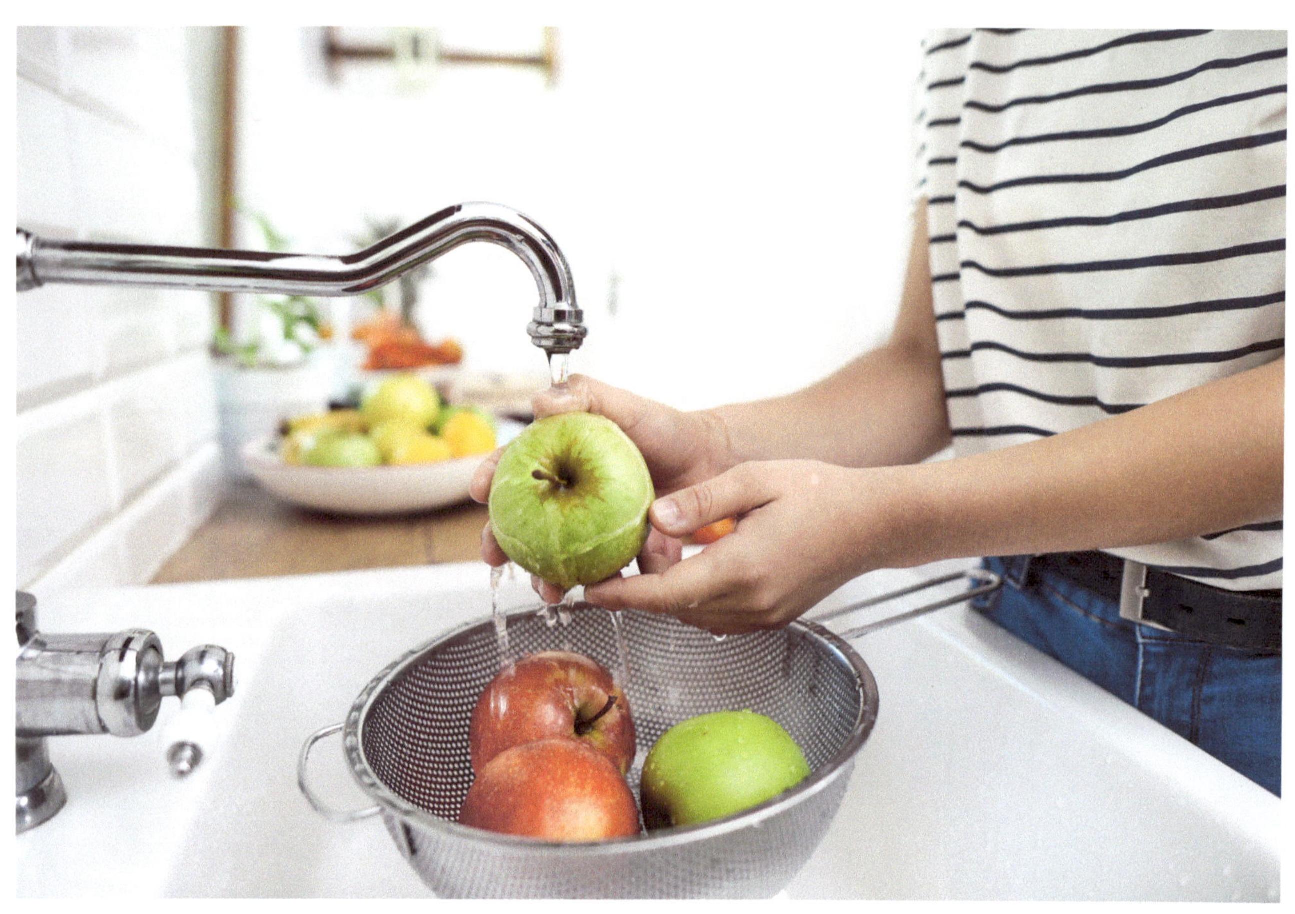

We wash the food.

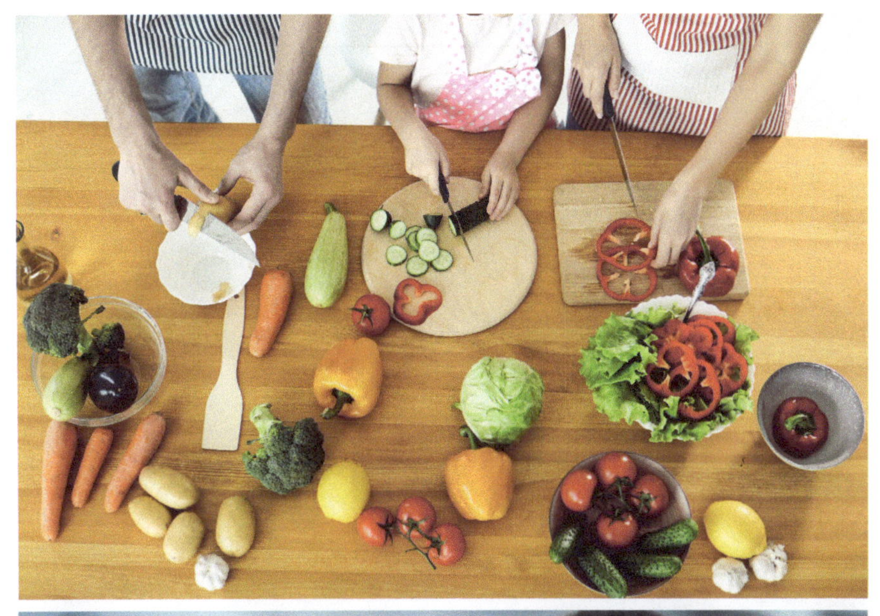

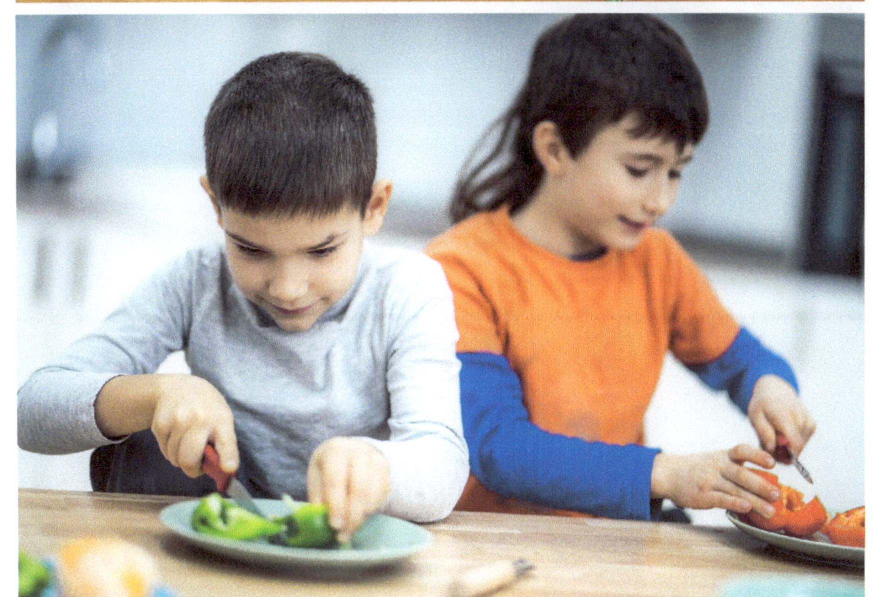

We cut the food.

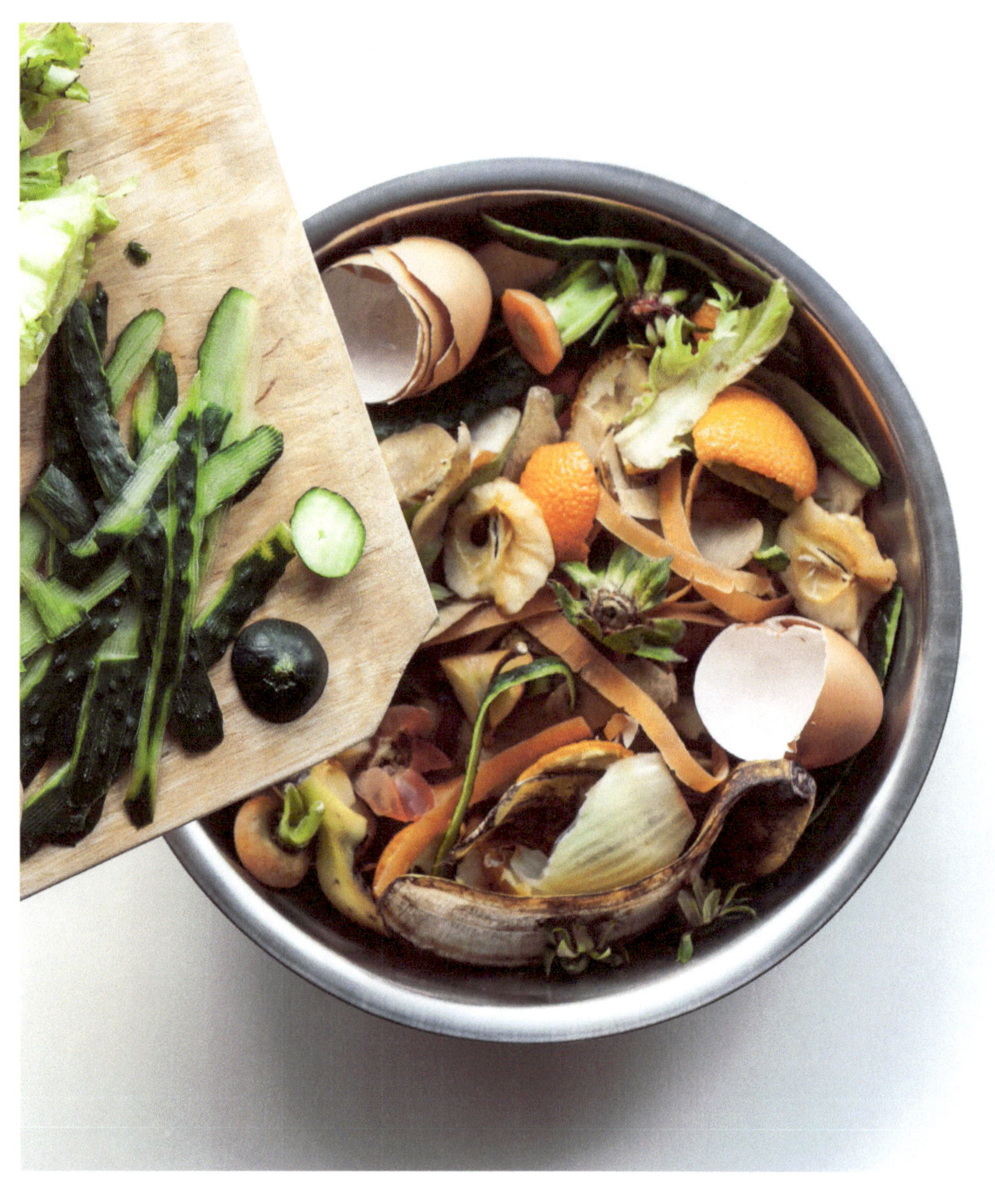

We add food scraps to the compost.

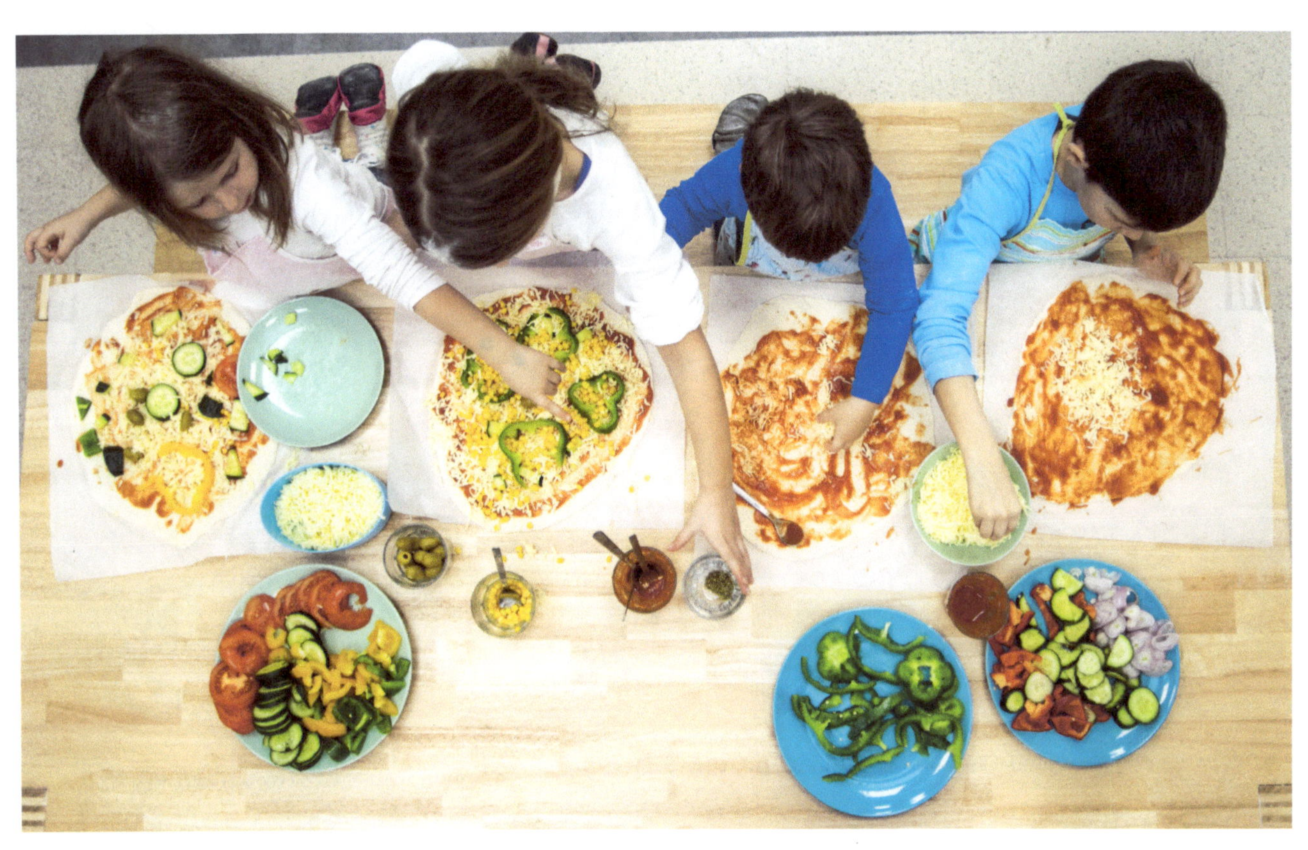

We cook the food.

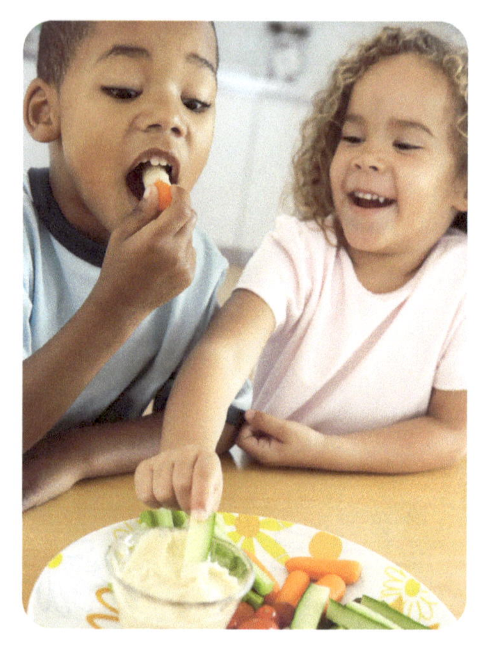

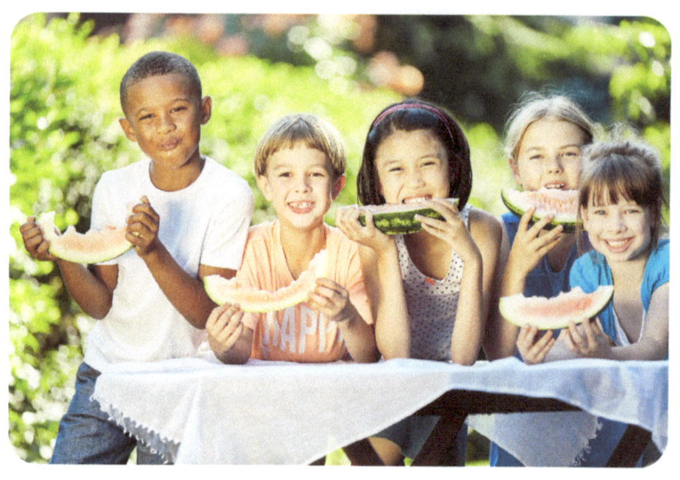

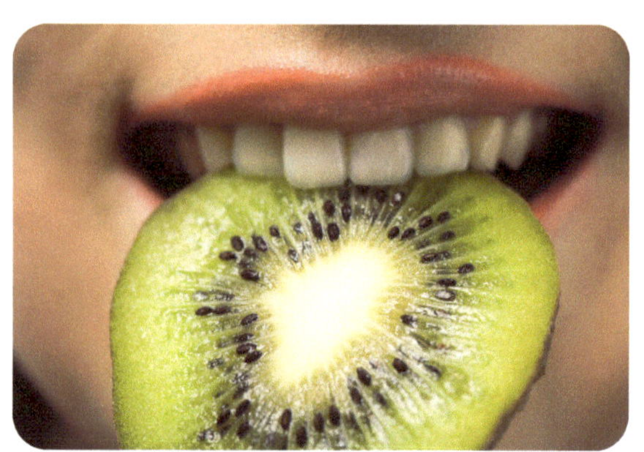

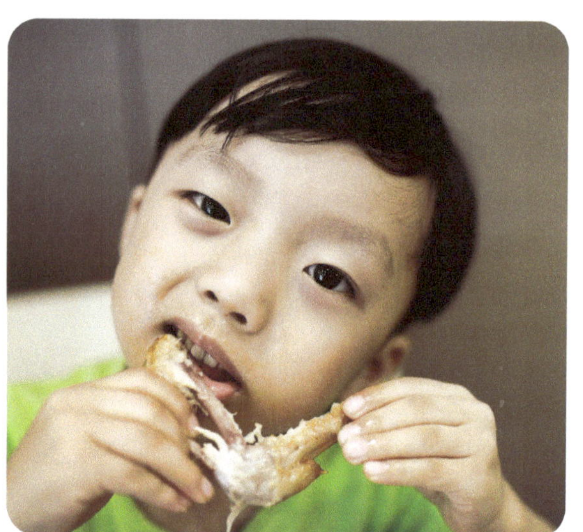

We eat the food.

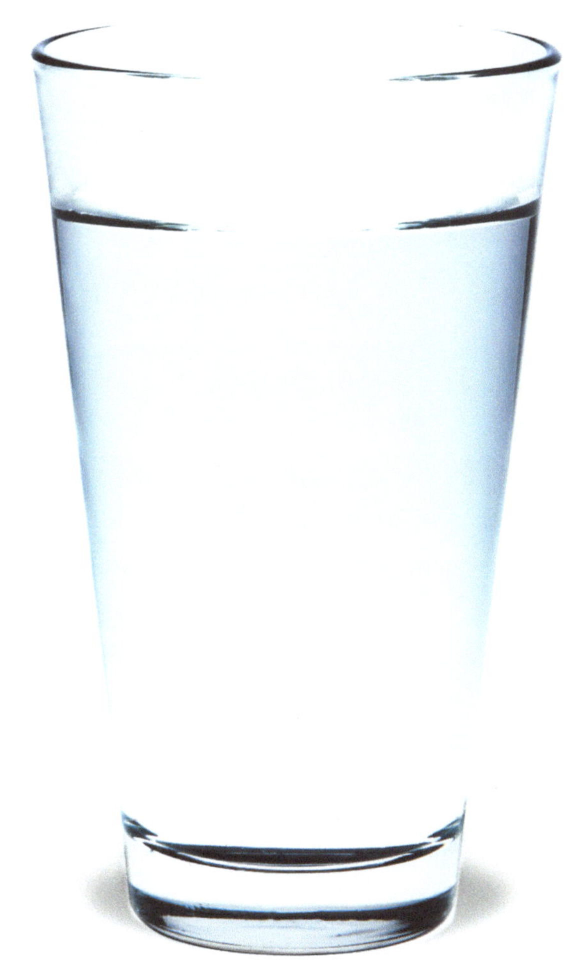

We drink eight glasses of water every day.

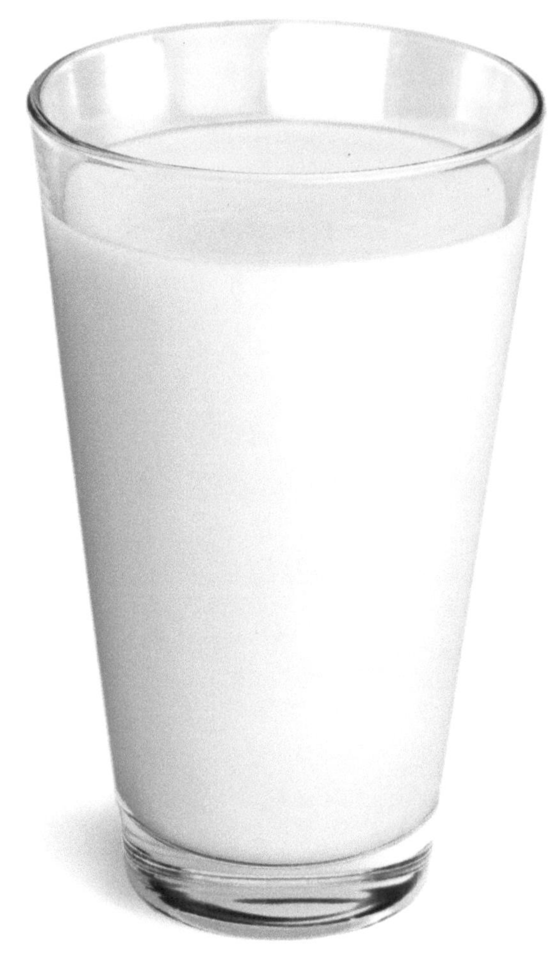

**We have a glass of milk.
Milk is dairy.**

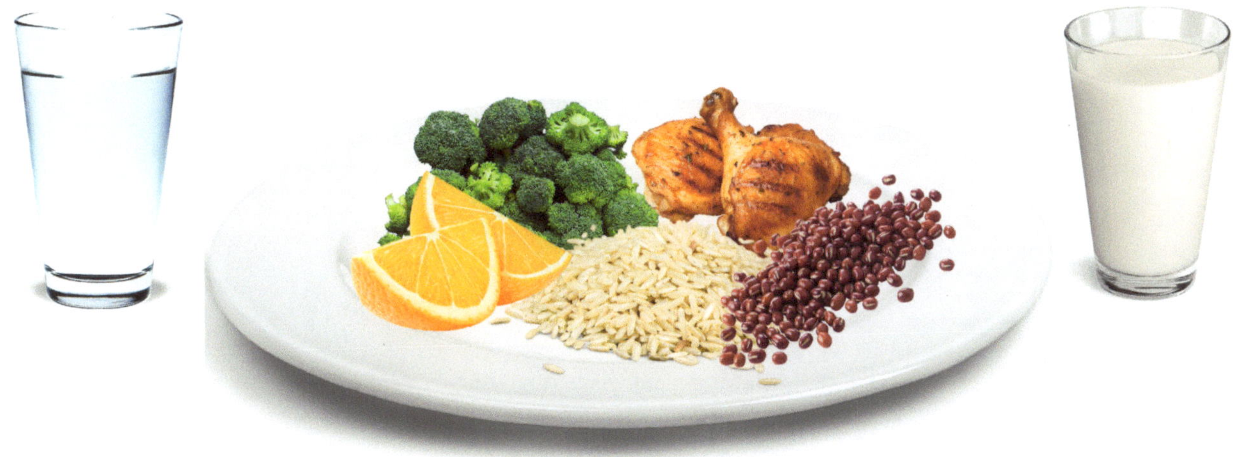

Look at our plate!

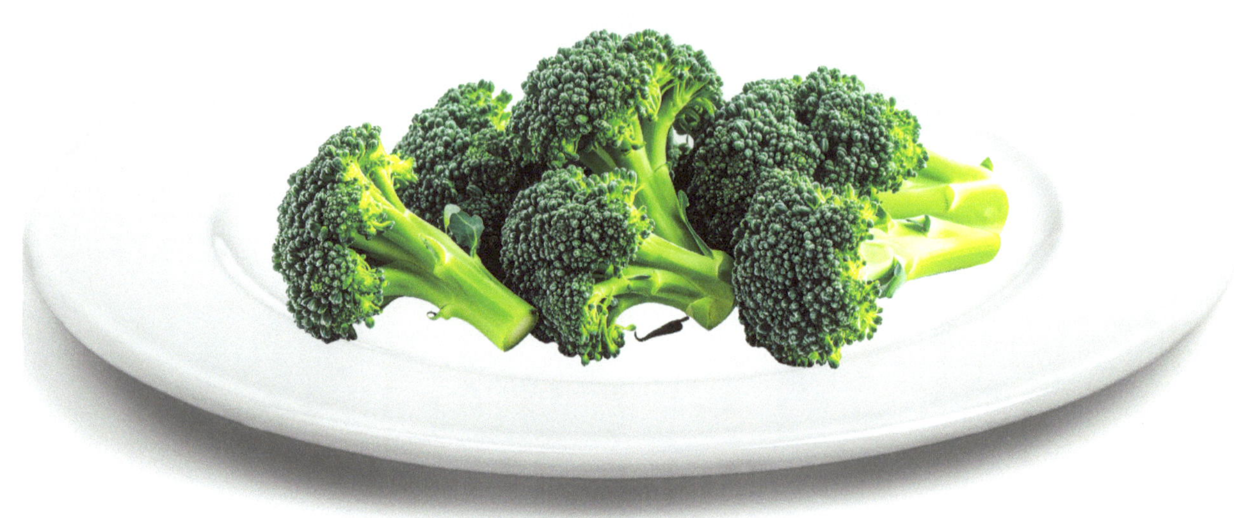

**We have broccoli on our plate.
Broccoli is a vegetable.**

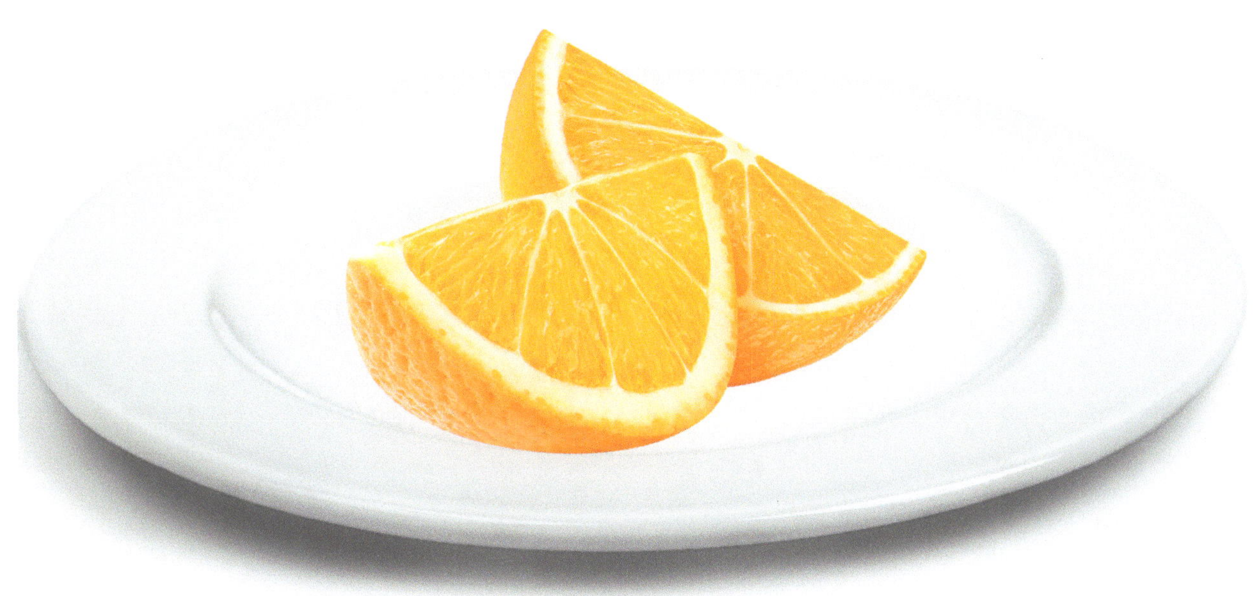

We have an orange on our plate.
Orange is a fruit.

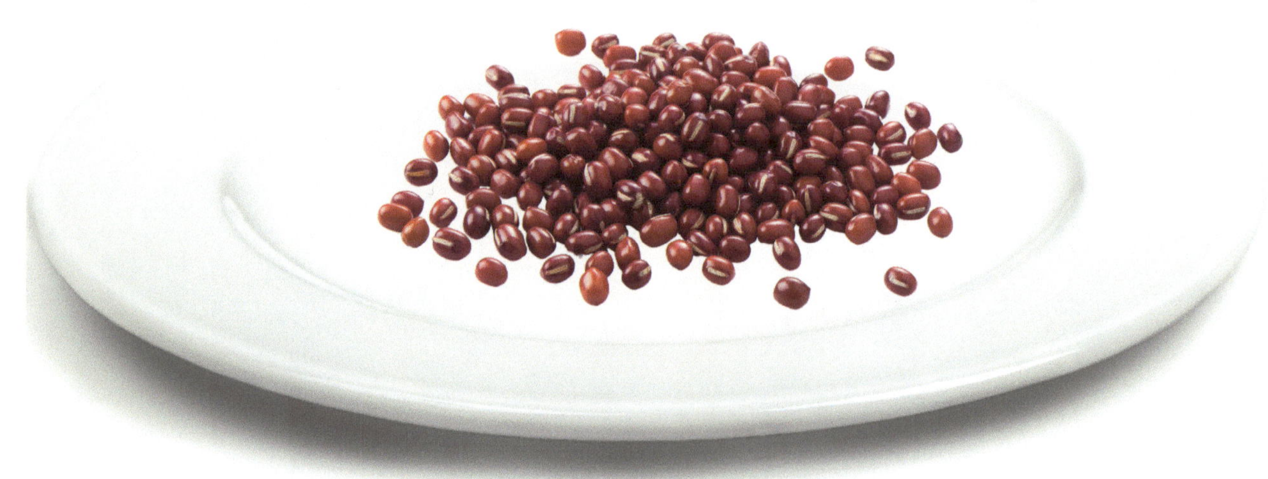

We have beans on our plate.
Beans are a good source of protein.

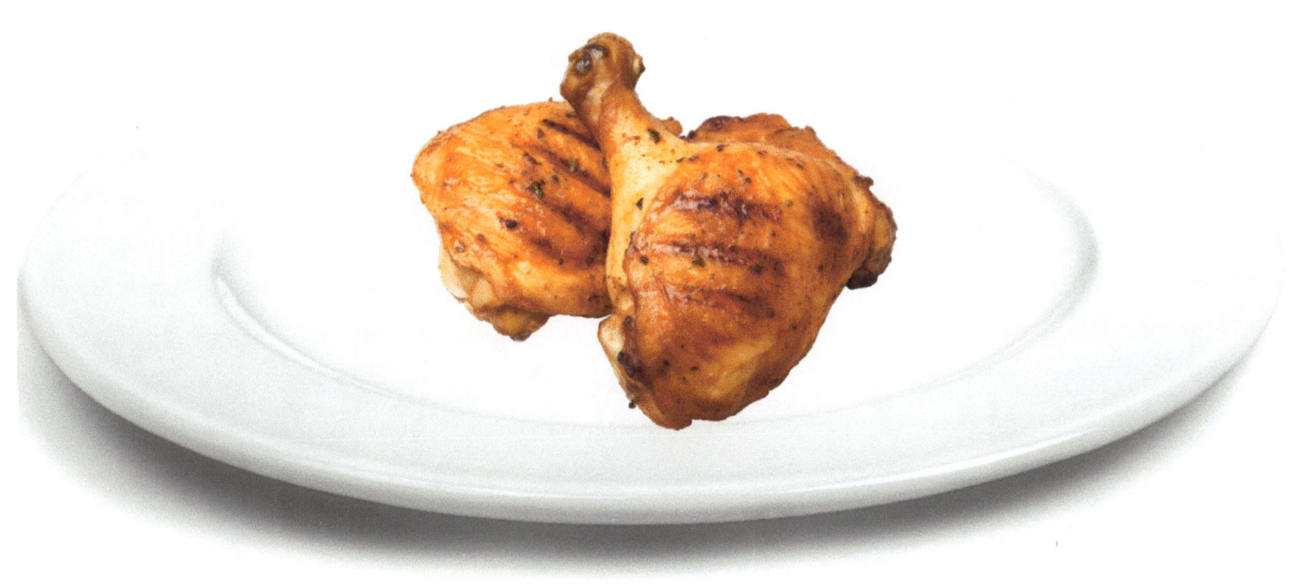

**We have chicken on our plate.
Chicken is a protein.**

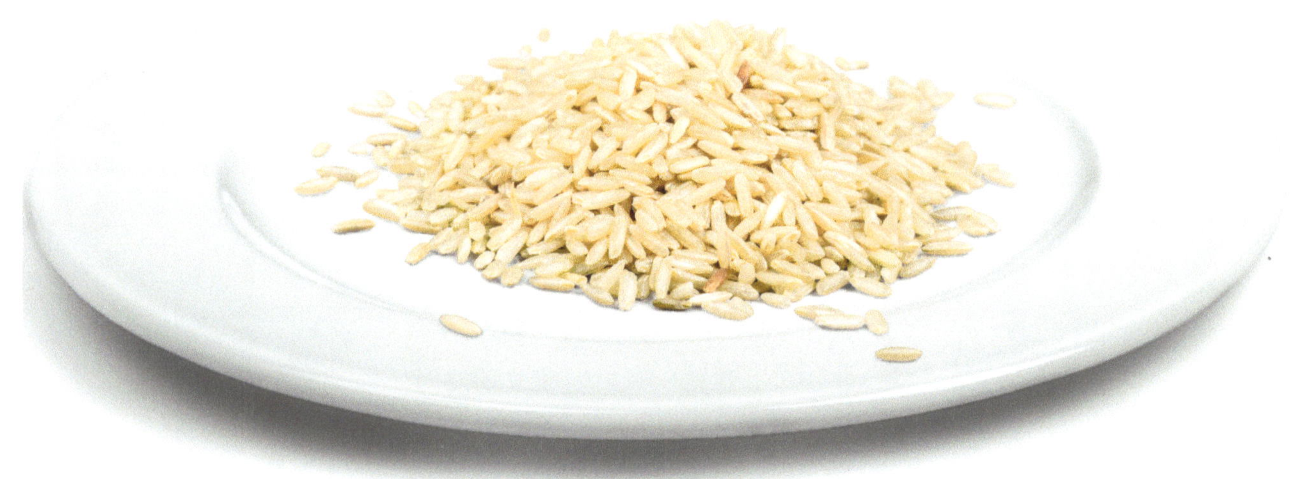

We have rice on our plate.
Rice is a grain.

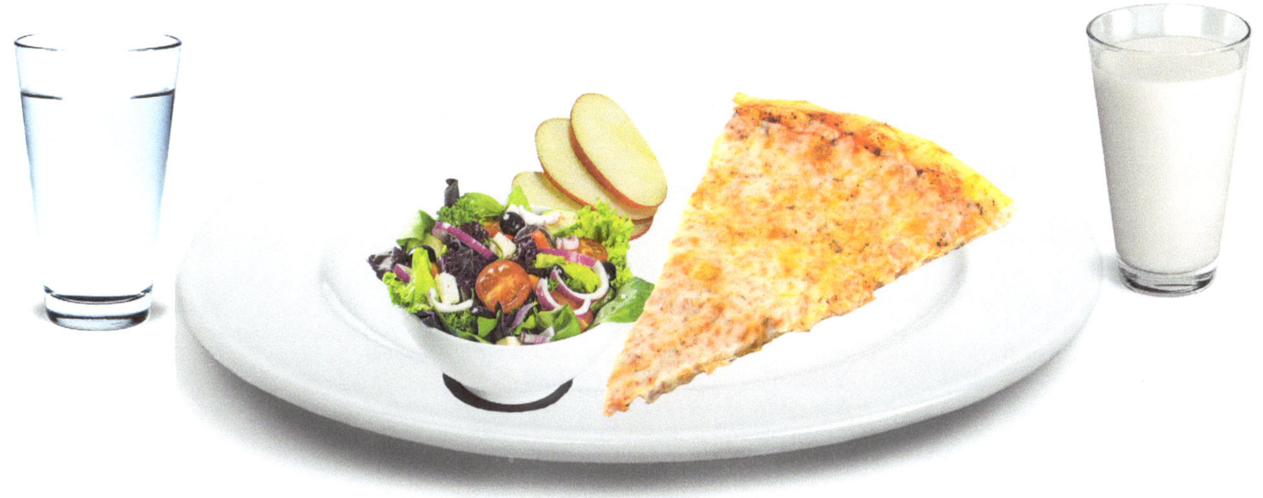

Look at our plate on Monday.

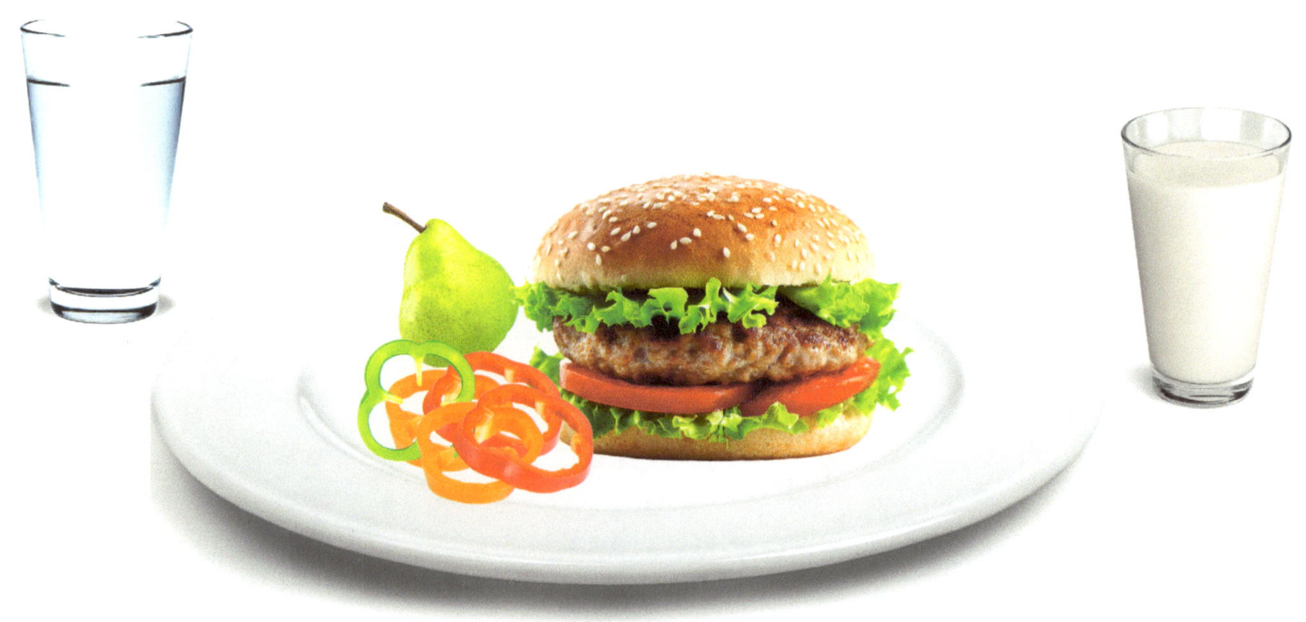

Look at our plate on Tuesday.

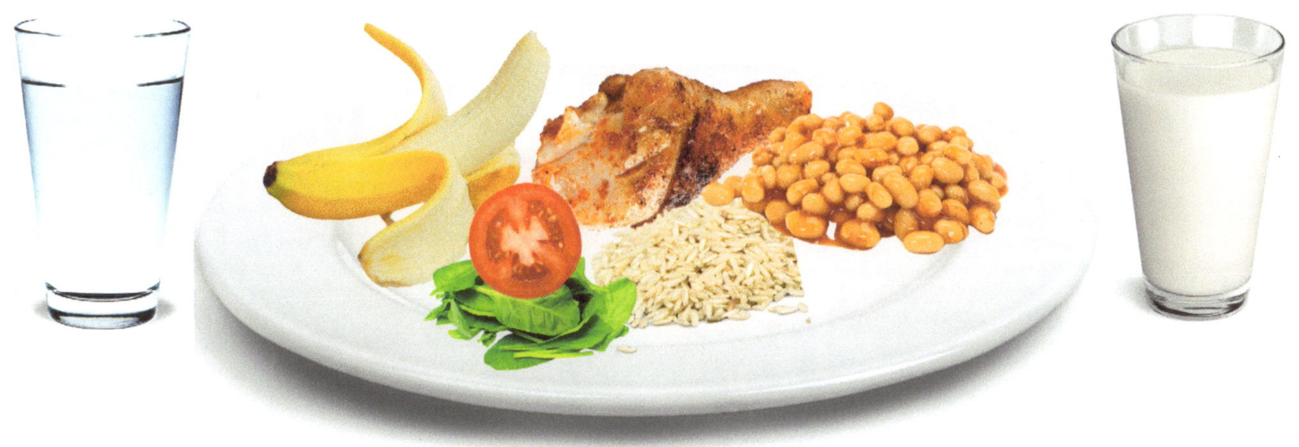

Look at our plate on Wednesday.

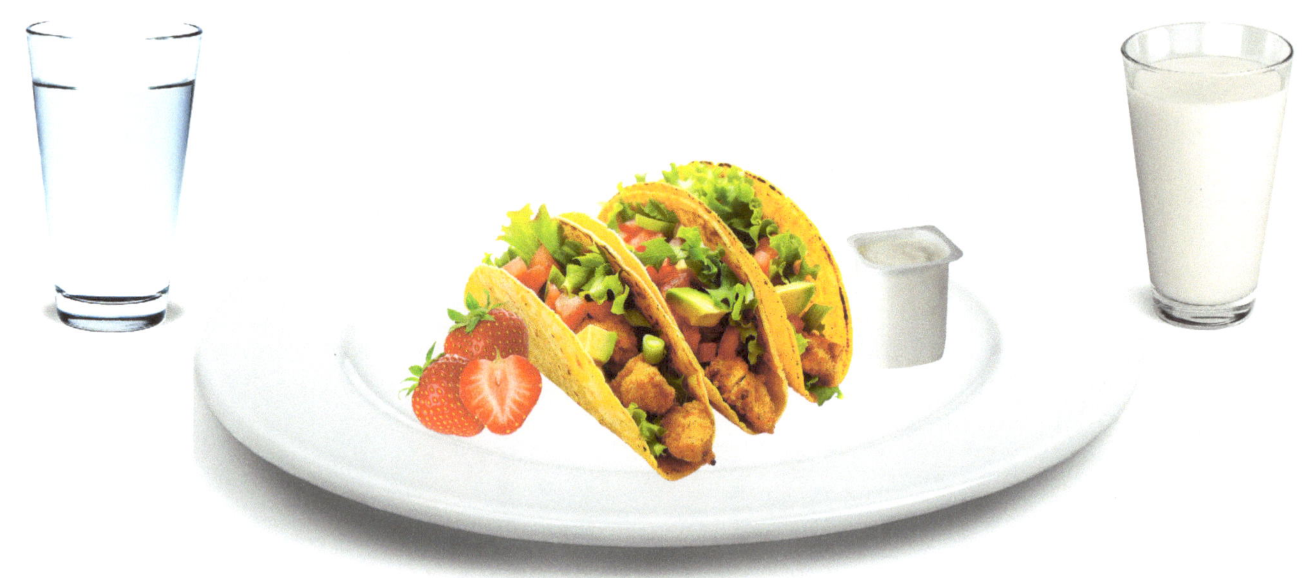

Look at our plate on Thursday.

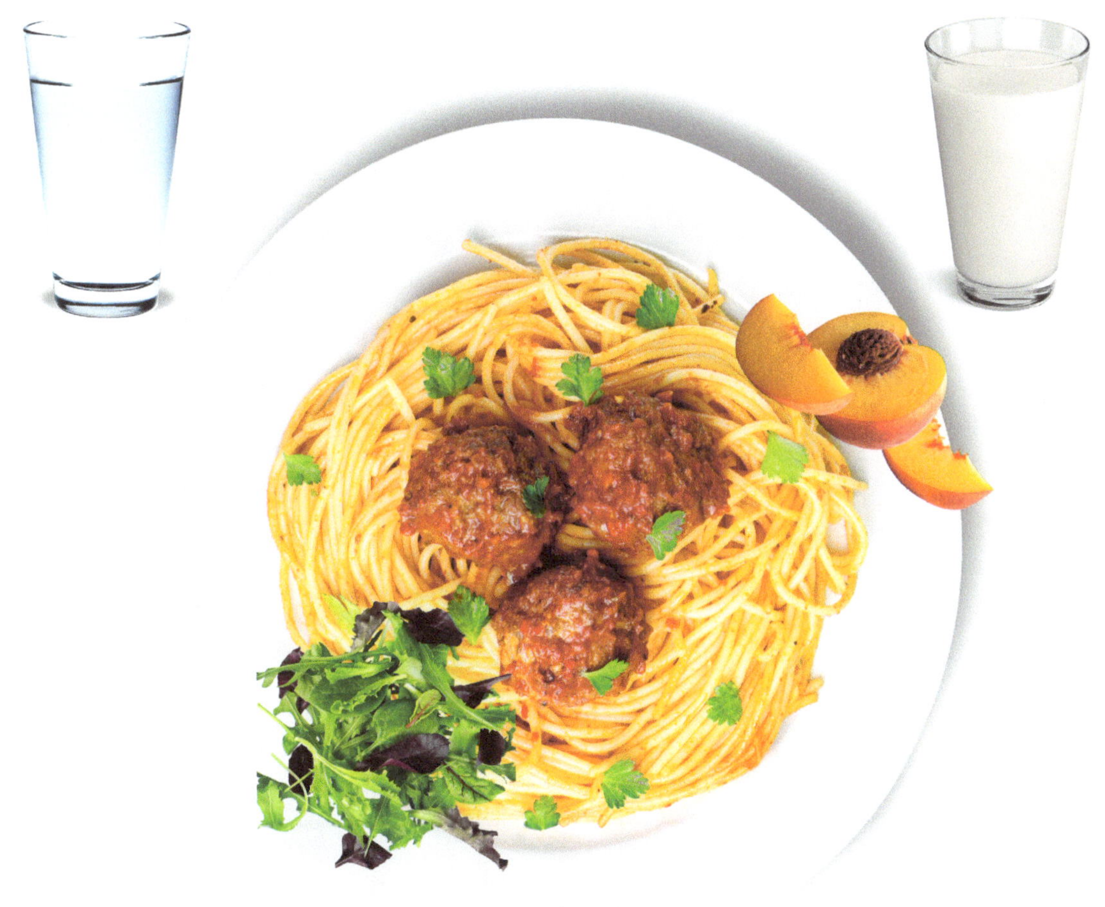

Look at my plate on Friday.

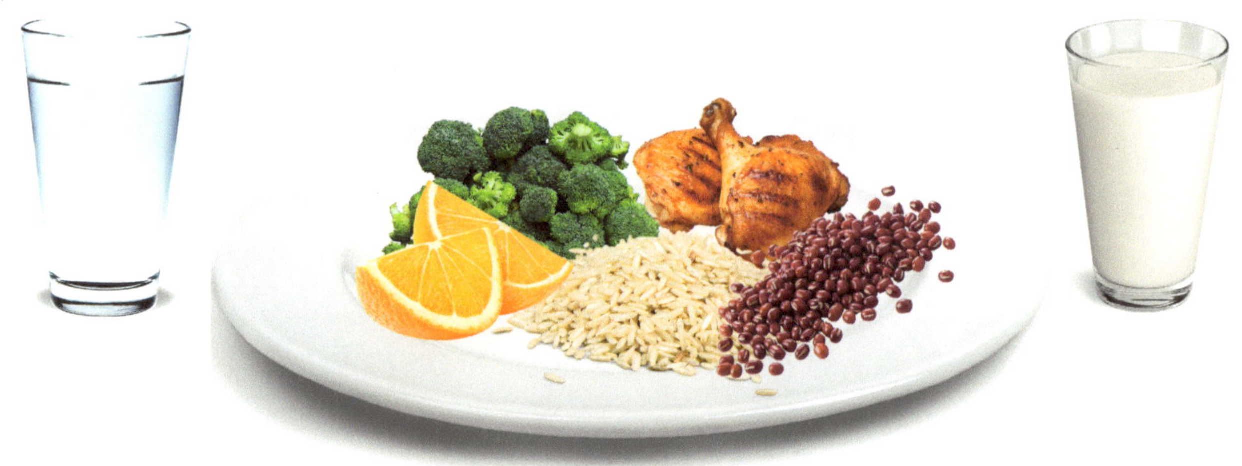

Look at our plate!

The students chant!

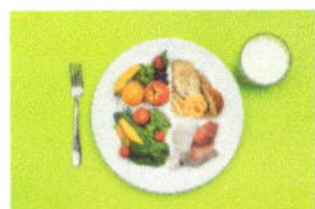

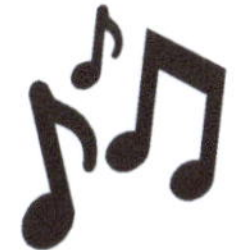

Do you know the five food groups?
The five food groups, the five food groups
Let us say the five food groups
Fruits, vegetables, grains, protein, and dairy
Yes, these are the five food groups!

Milk is dairy
Chicken is a protein
Orange is a fruit
Broccoli is a vegetable
Rice is a grain
Yes, these are the five food groups!
All on my plate!

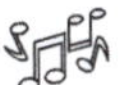

Which food group is your favorite?
is your favorite, is your favorite
[Insert Name/Group] is my favorite,
Is my favorite, is my favorite!
[Insert Name/Group] is my favorite,
It makes me feel so good!

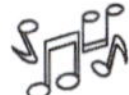

Fruits, vegetables, grains,
Protein, and dairy!
Fruits, vegetables, grains,
Protein, and dairy!
Yes, these are the five food groups,
Let's eat them every day!

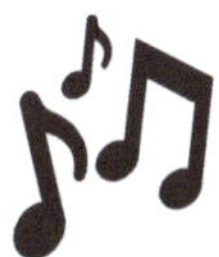

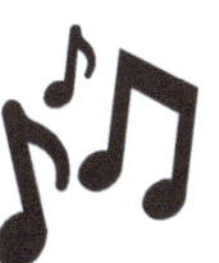

What is on your plate?
It's your turn to make your plate!

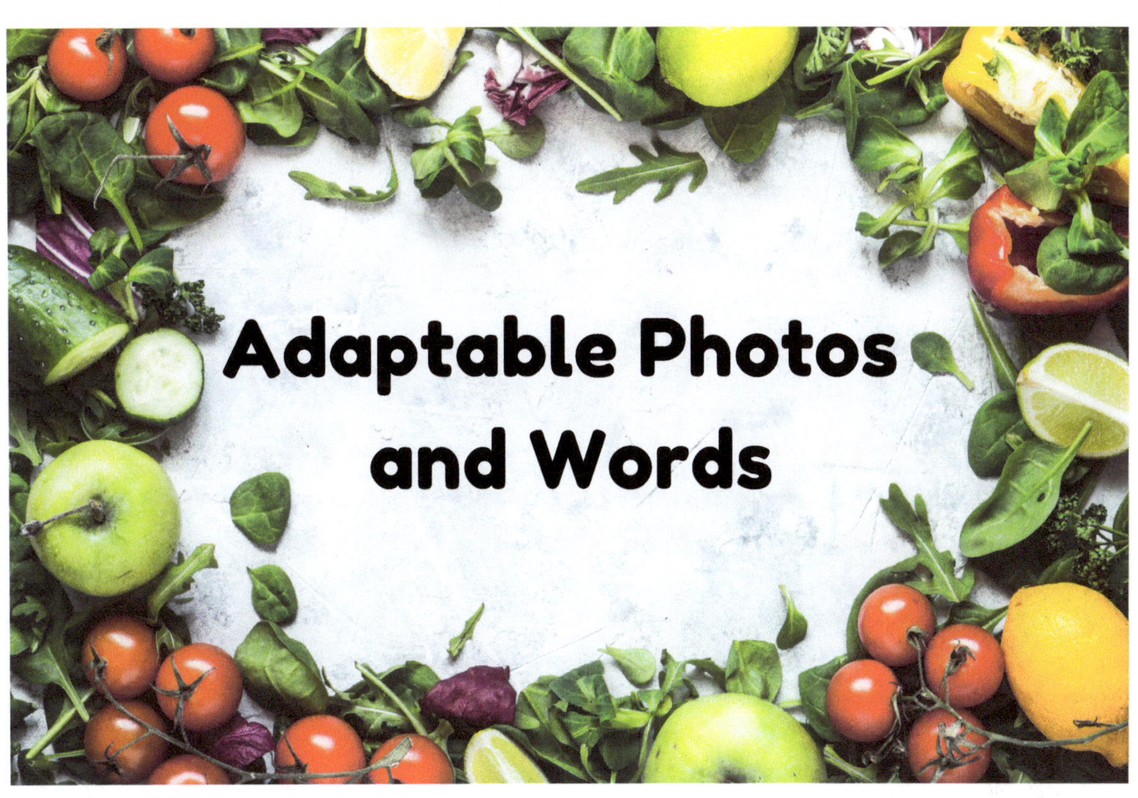
Adaptable Photos
and Words

Adaptable Photos and Words

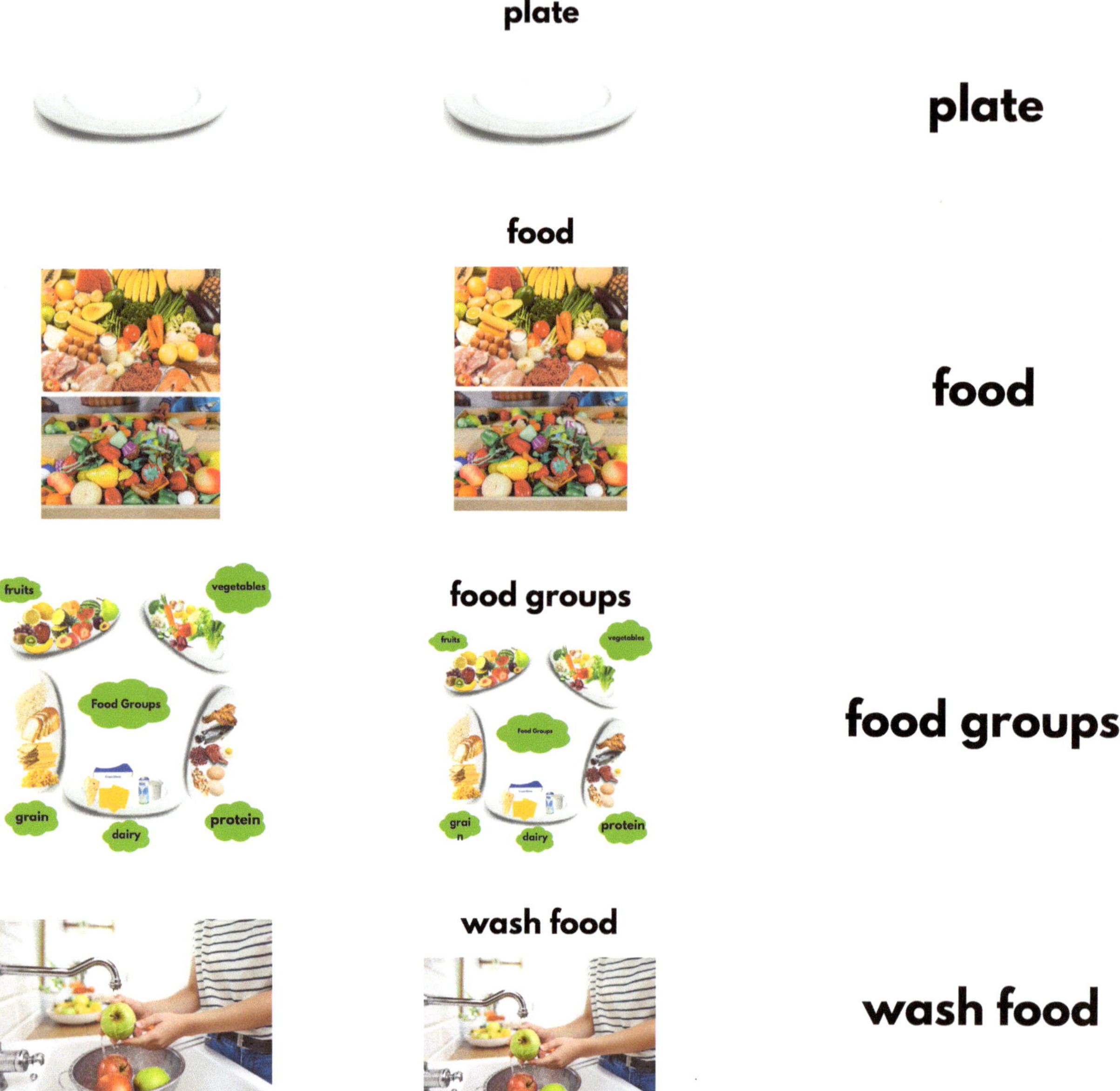

Adaptable Photos and Words

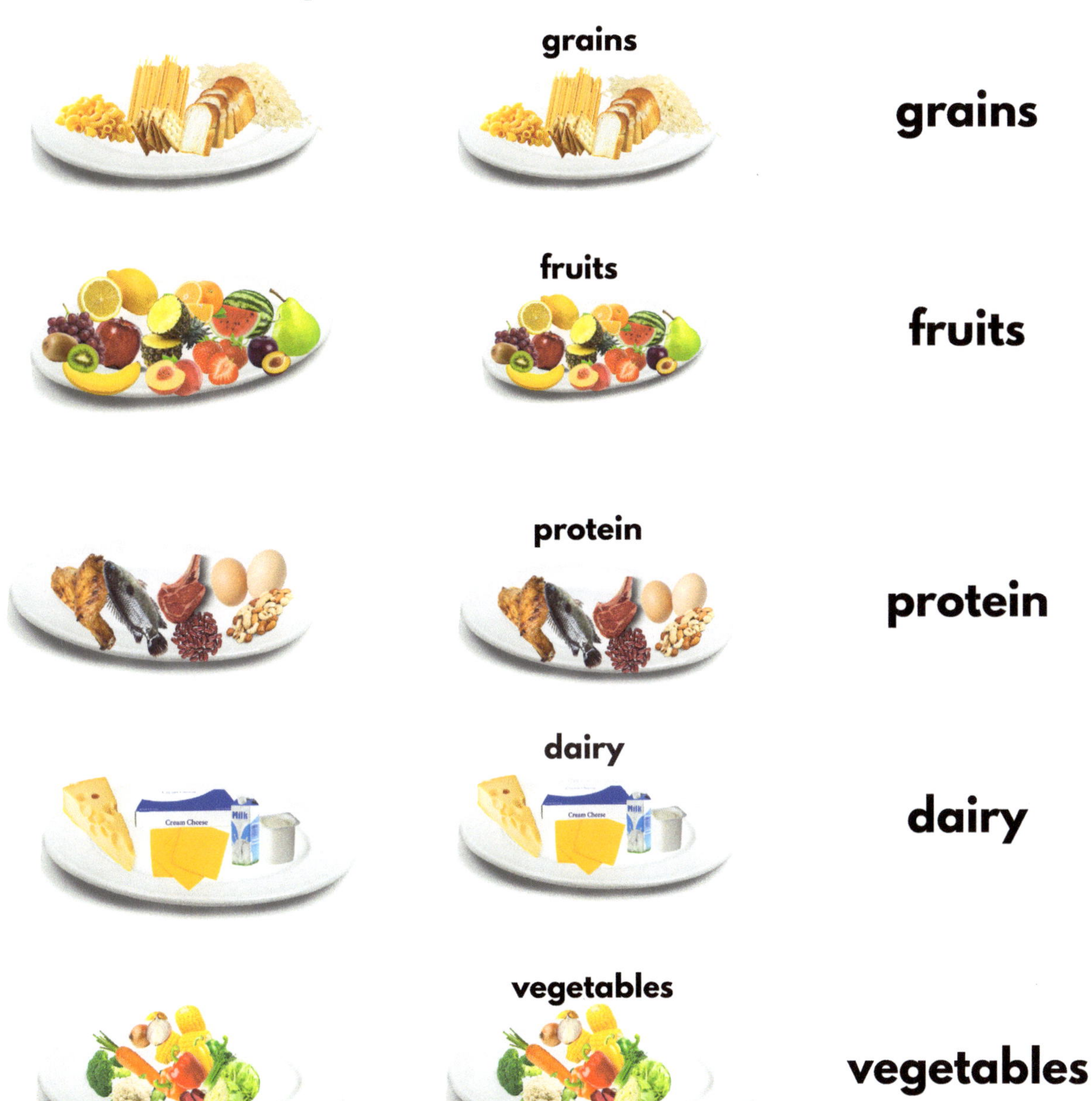

Adaptable Photos and Words

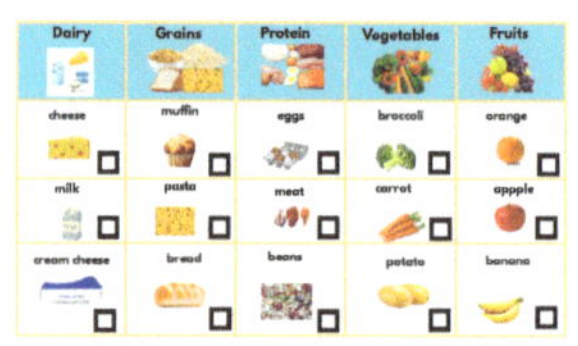

Dairy	Grains	Protein	Vegetables	Fruits
cheese	muffin	eggs	broccoli	orange
milk	pasta	meat	carrot	appple
cream cheese	bread	beans	potato	banana

Grocery List

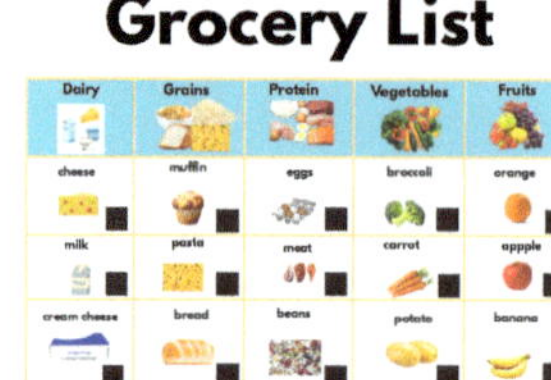

Dairy	Grains	Protein	Vegetables	Fruits
cheese	muffin	eggs	broccoli	orange
milk	pasta	meat	carrot	appple
cream cheese	bread	beans	potato	banana

Grocery List

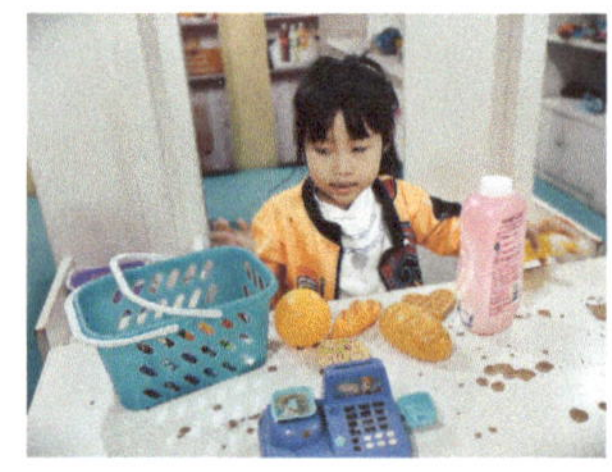

Grocery Store

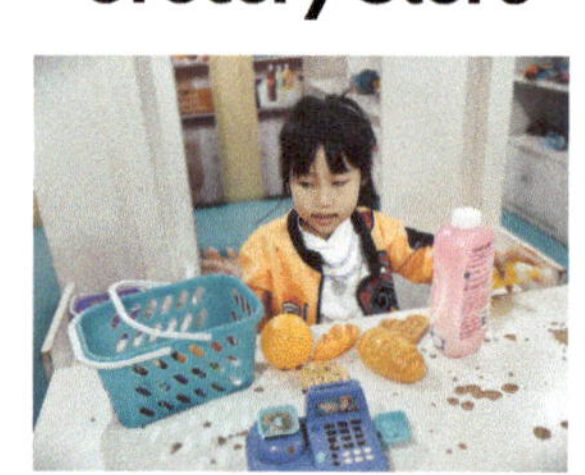

Grocery Store

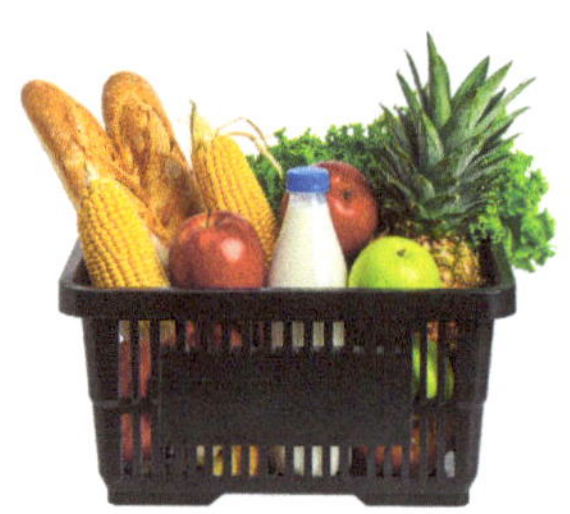

shop

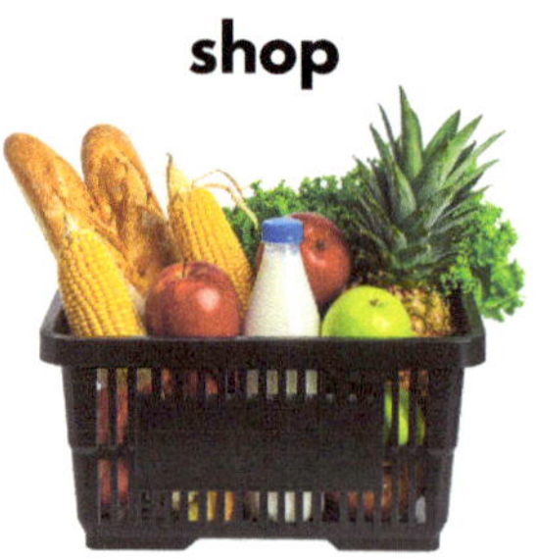

shop

Adaptable Photos and Words

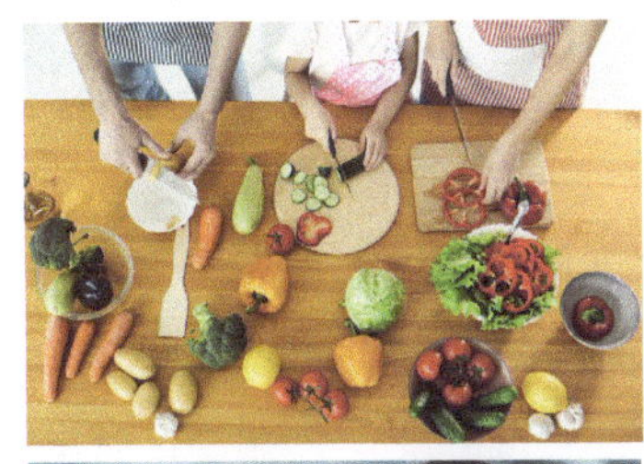

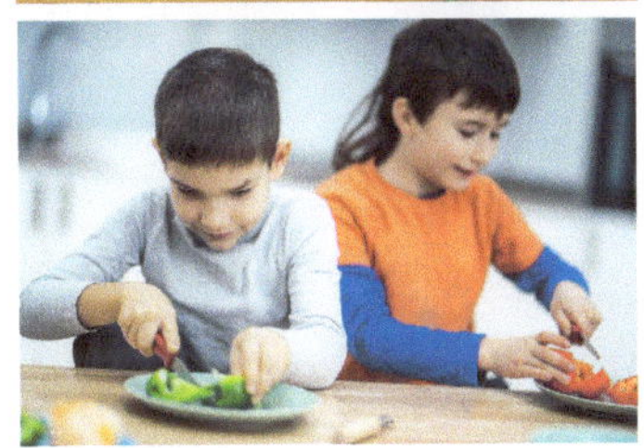

cut food

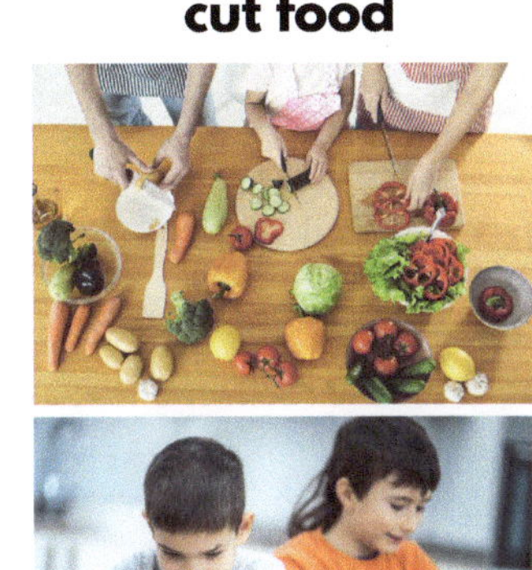

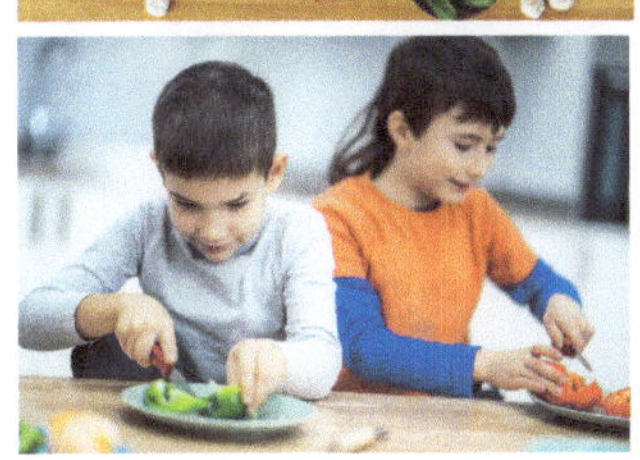

cut food

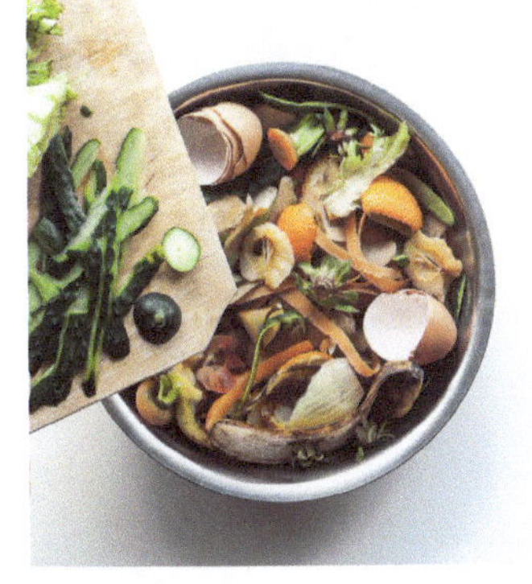

food scraps

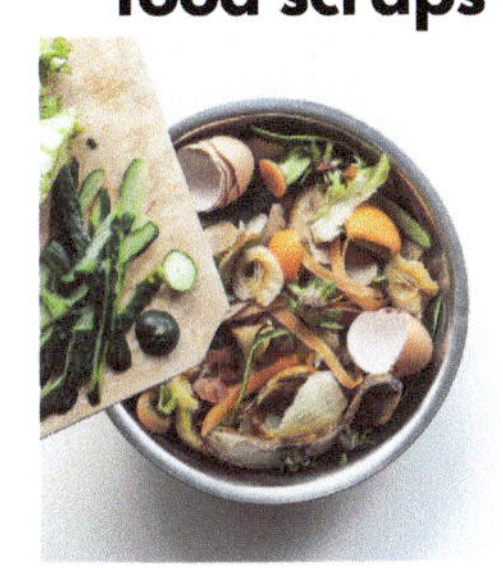

food scraps

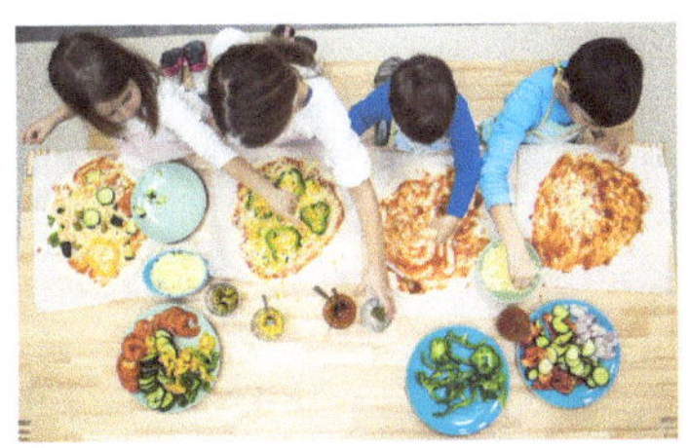

cook

cook

Adaptable Photos and Words

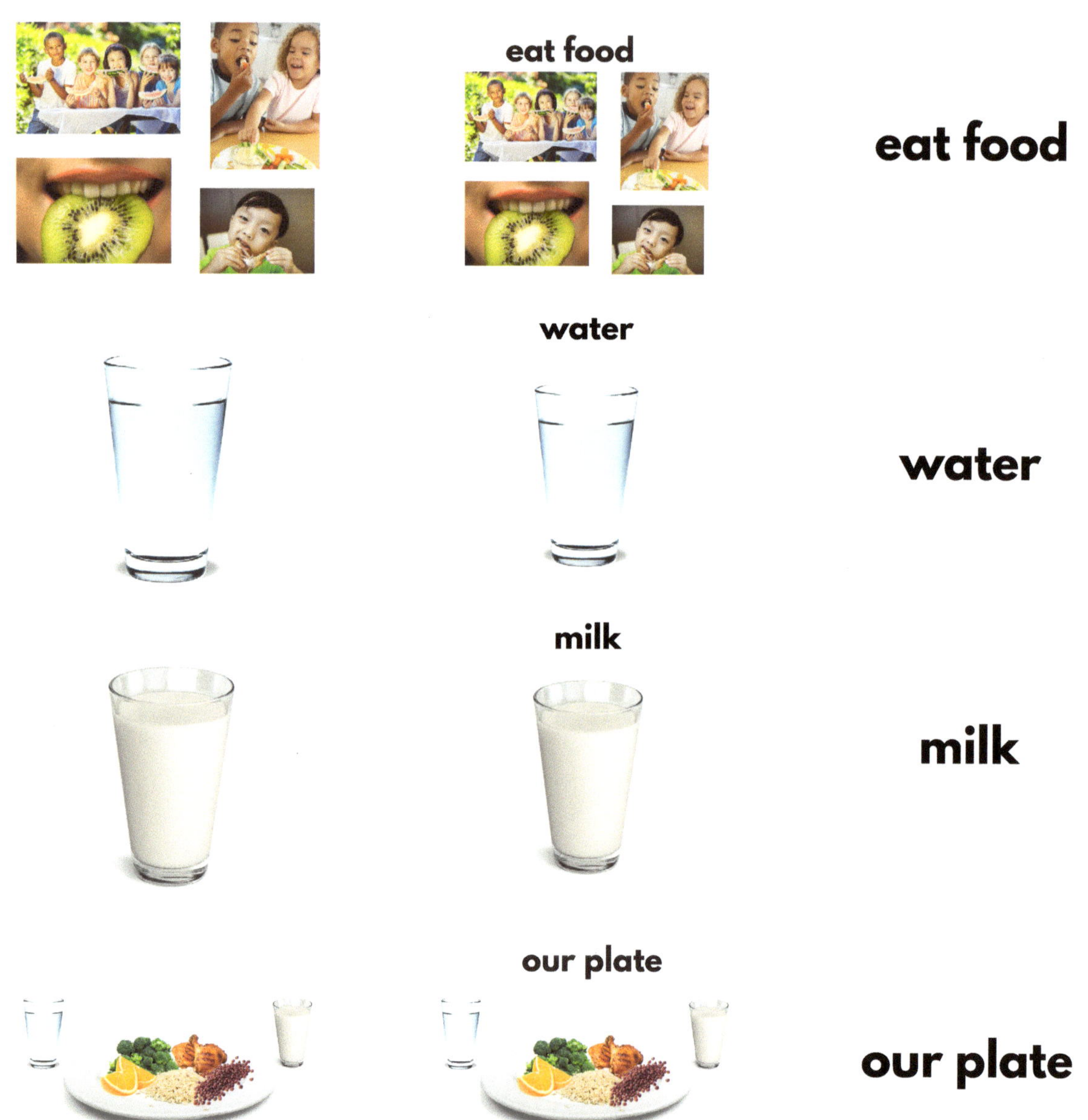

Adaptable Photos and Words

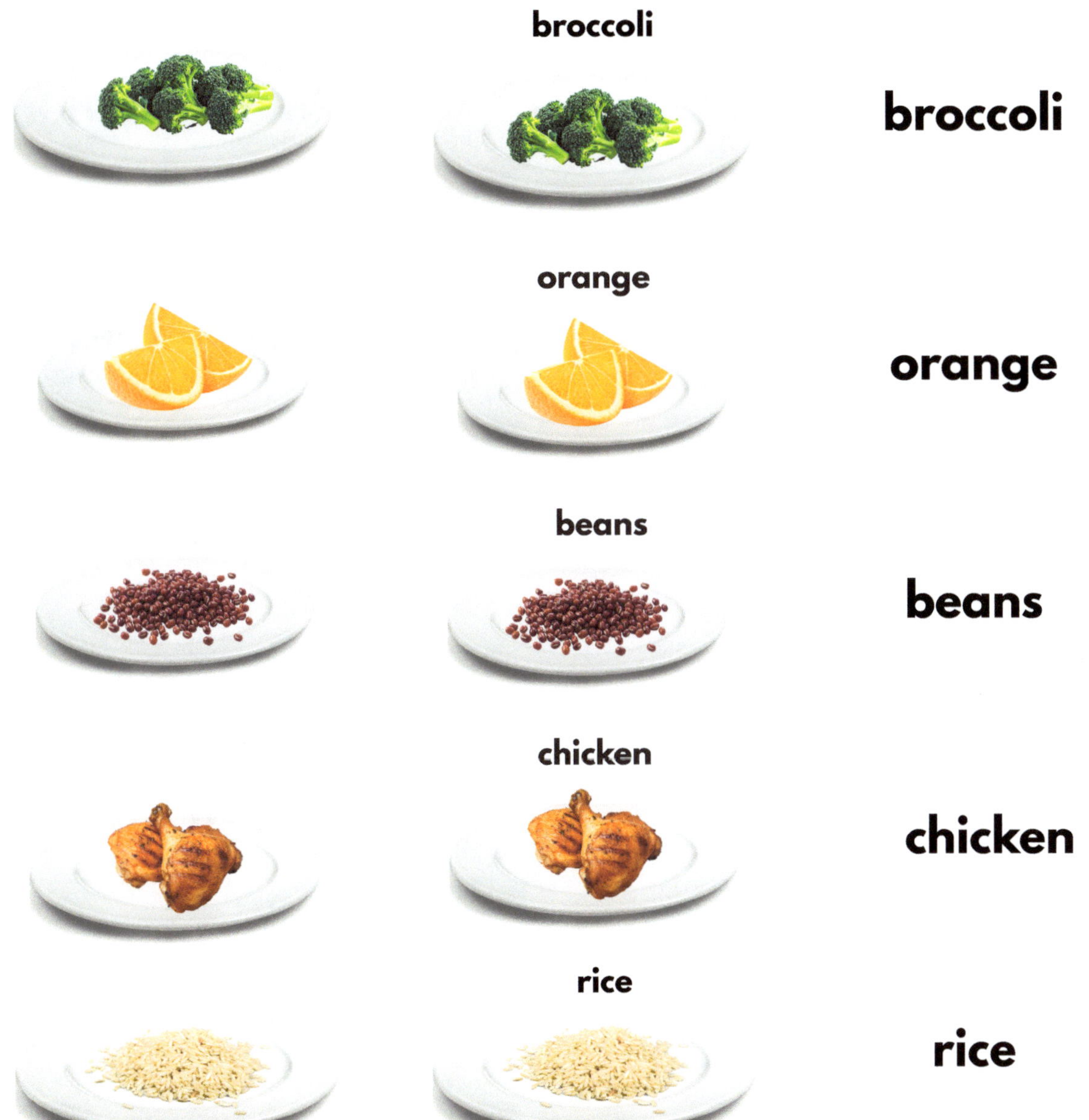

Adaptable Photos and Words

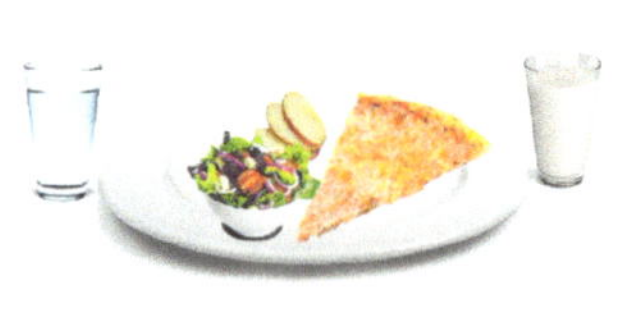

plate on Monday

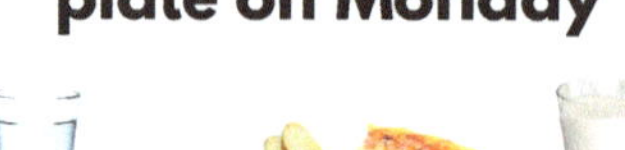

plate on Monday

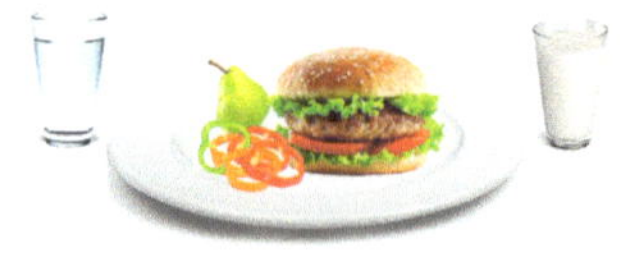

plate on Tuesday

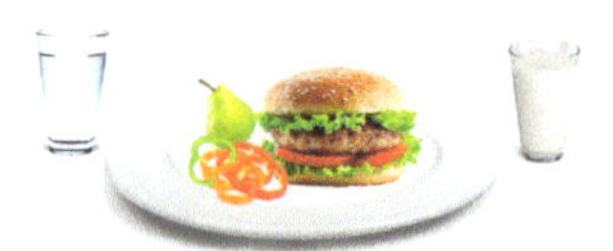

plate on Tuesday

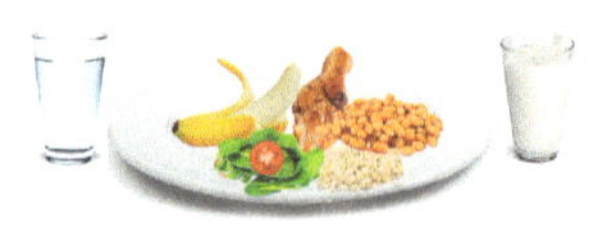

plate on Wednesday

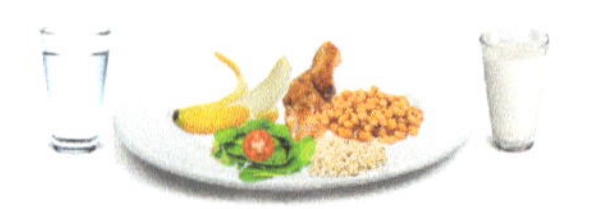

plate on Wednesday

plate on Thursday

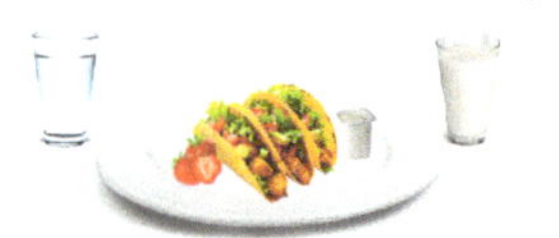

plate on Thursday

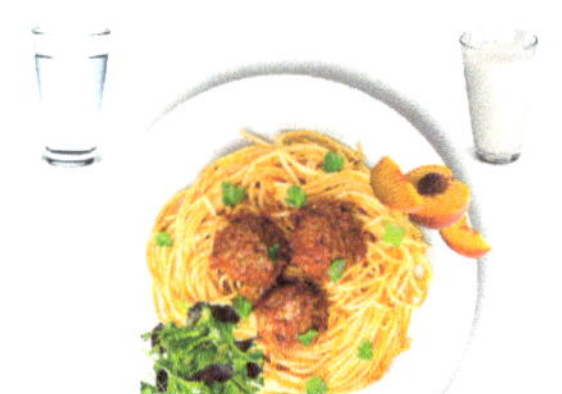

plate on Friday

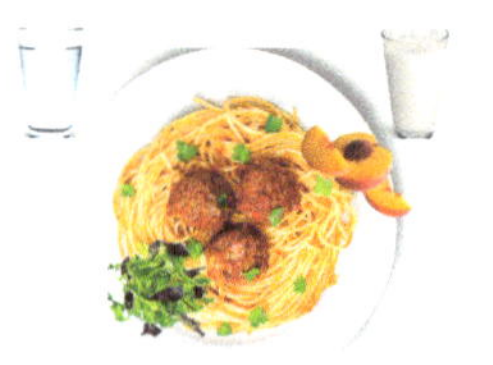

plate on Friday

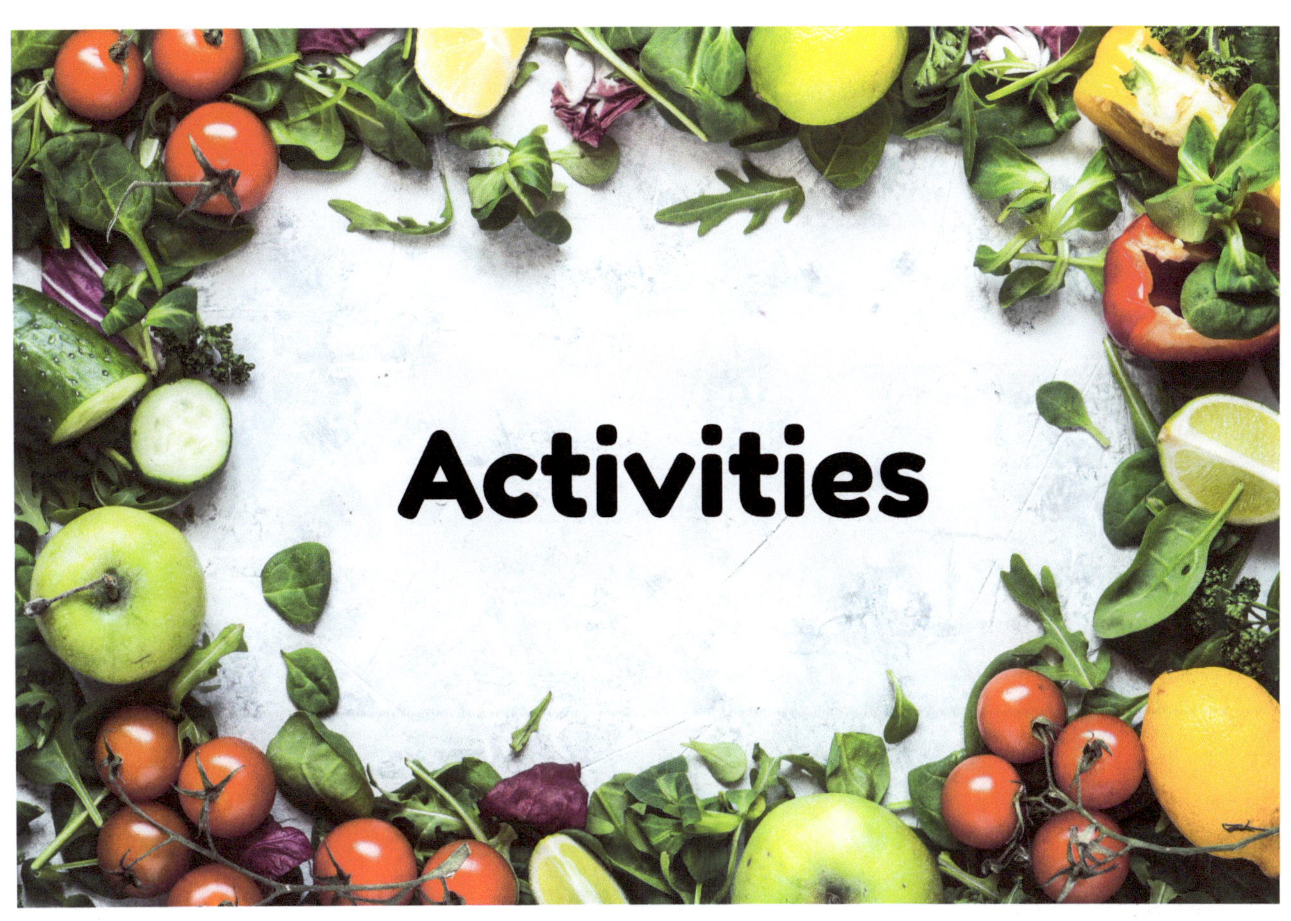
Activities

Label the food groups

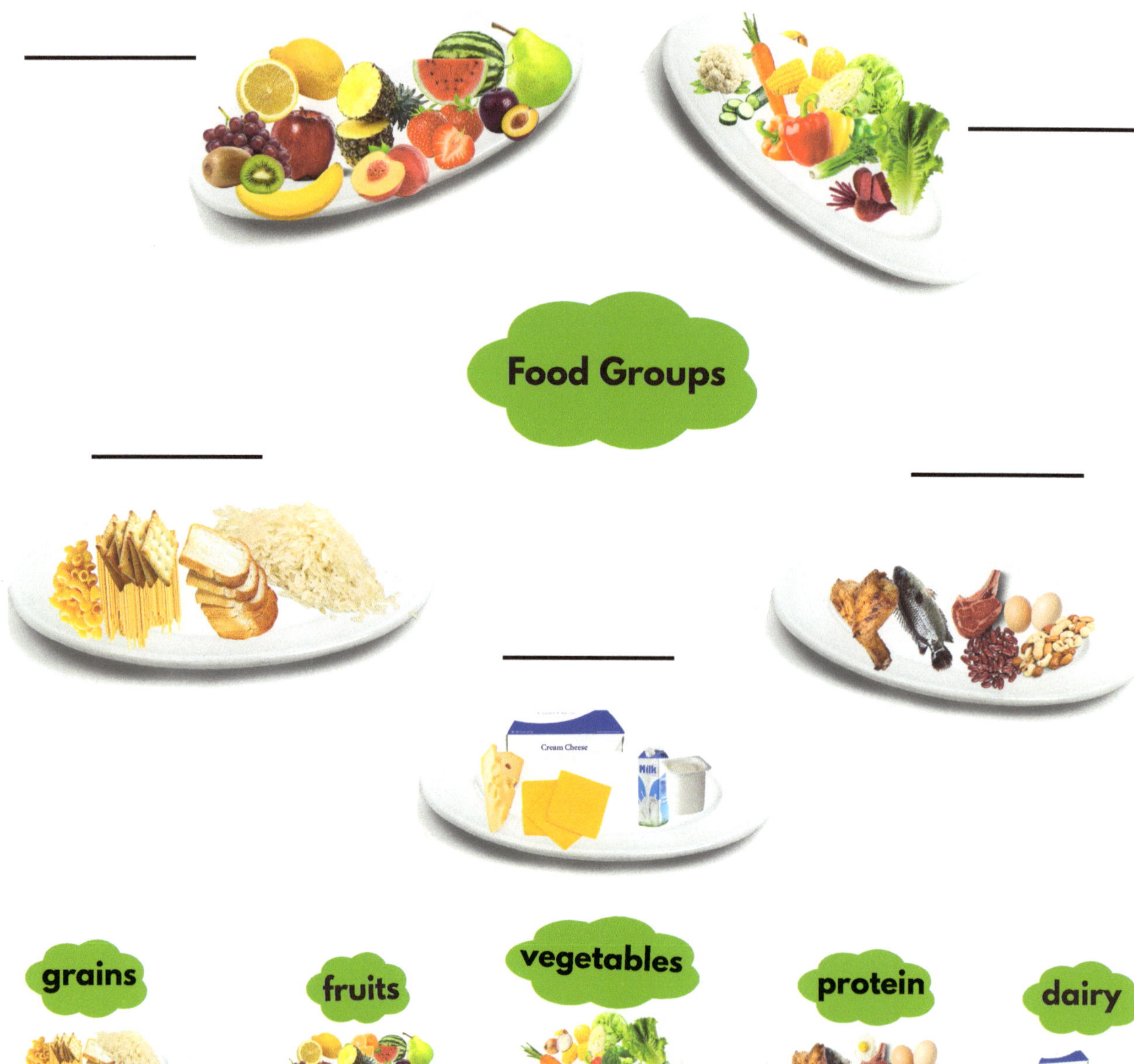

grains fruits vegetables protein dairy

Label the food groups

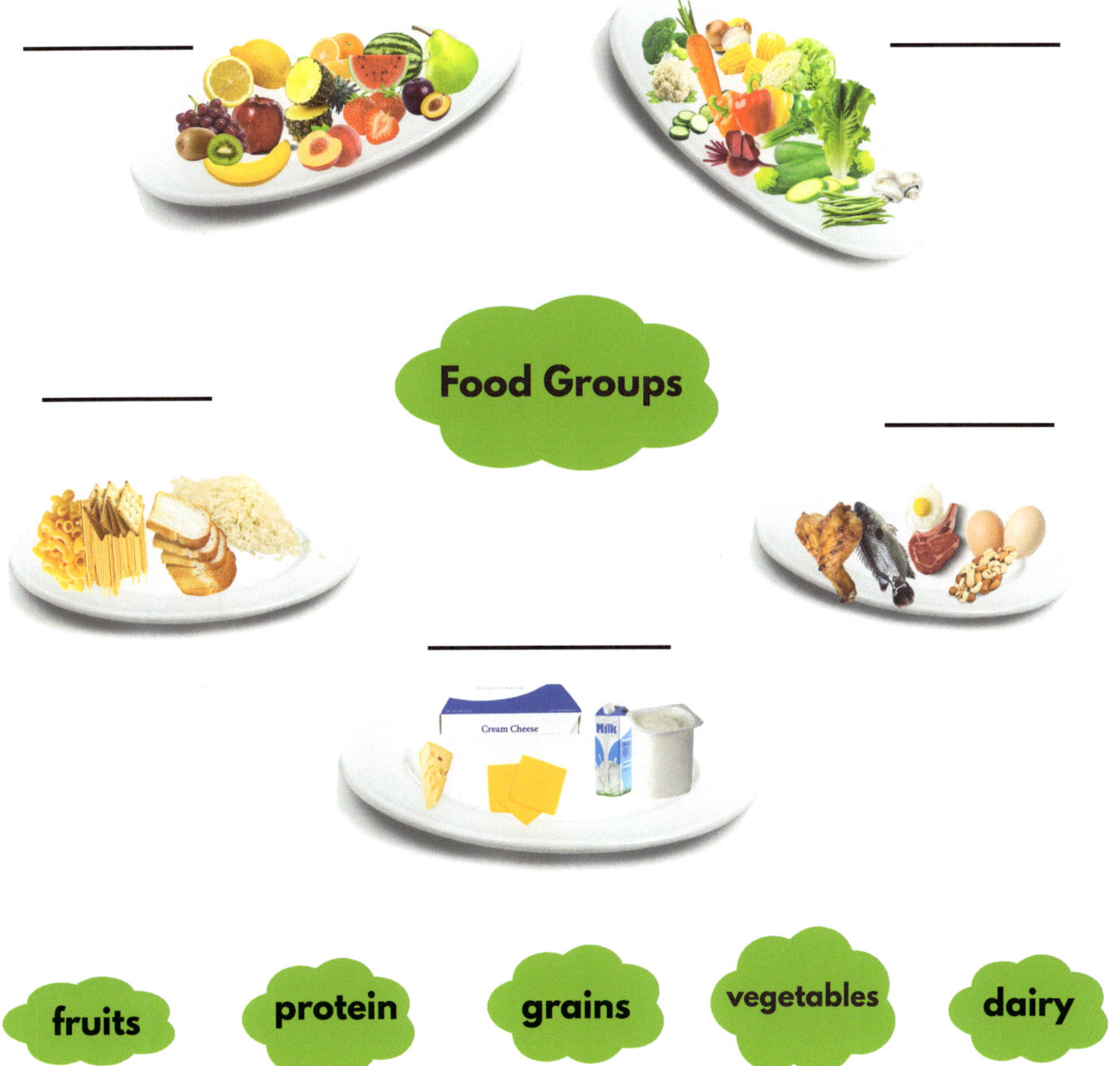

fruits

protein

grains

vegetables

dairy

Match the food to the correct food group

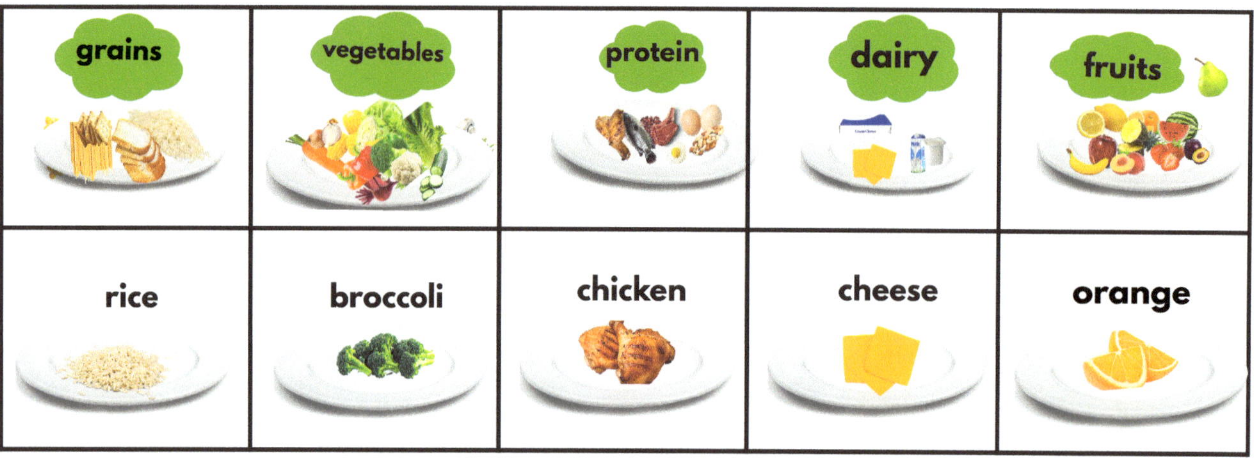

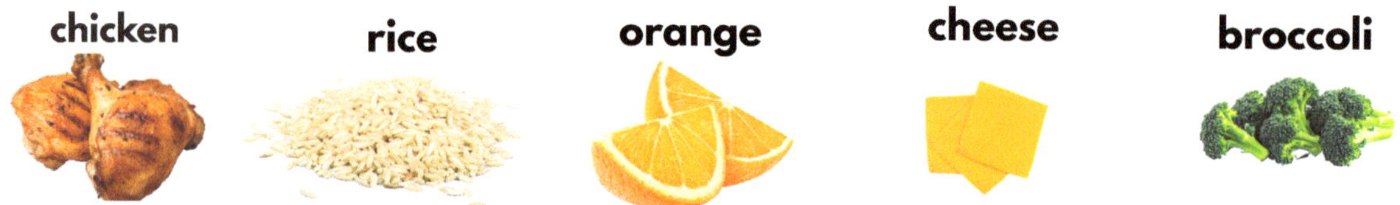

Match the food to the correct food group

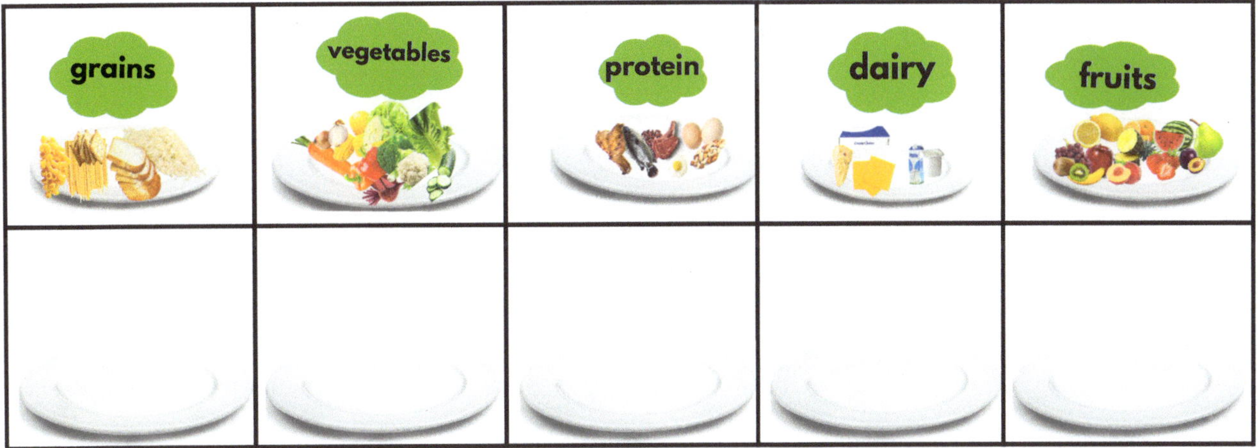

chicken

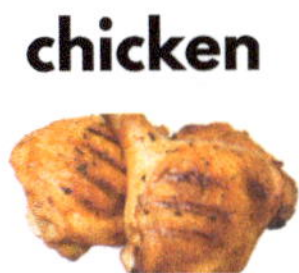

rice

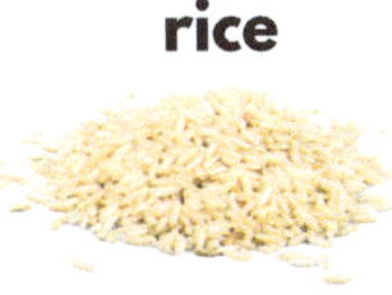

orange

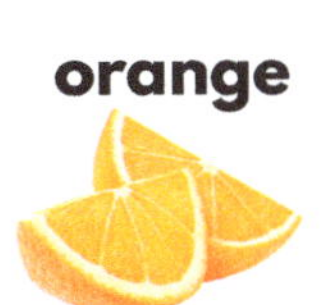

cheese

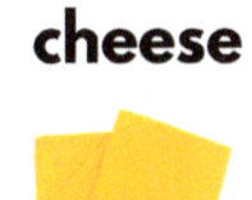

broccoli

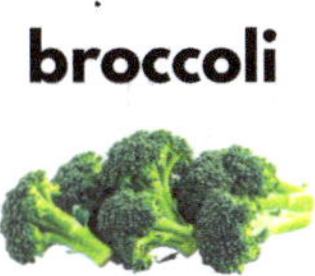

Write your name or put your picture on the chart to show your favorite food group

grains 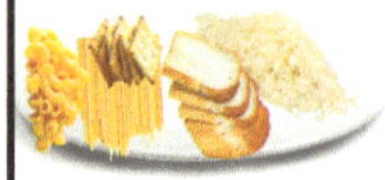	vegetables 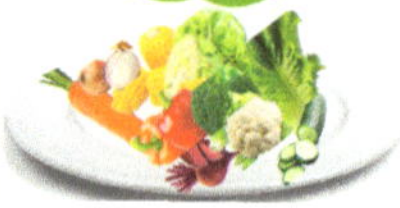	protein 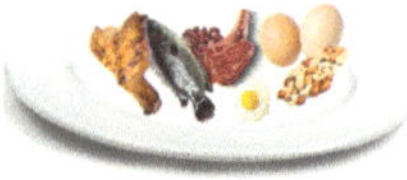	dairy 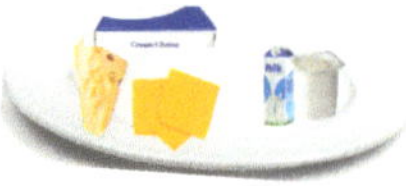	fruits 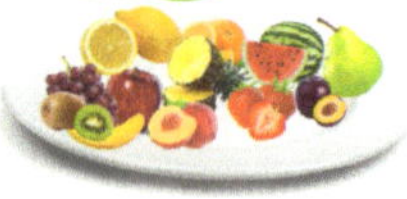

Look at Our Plate

A Balanced Meal!

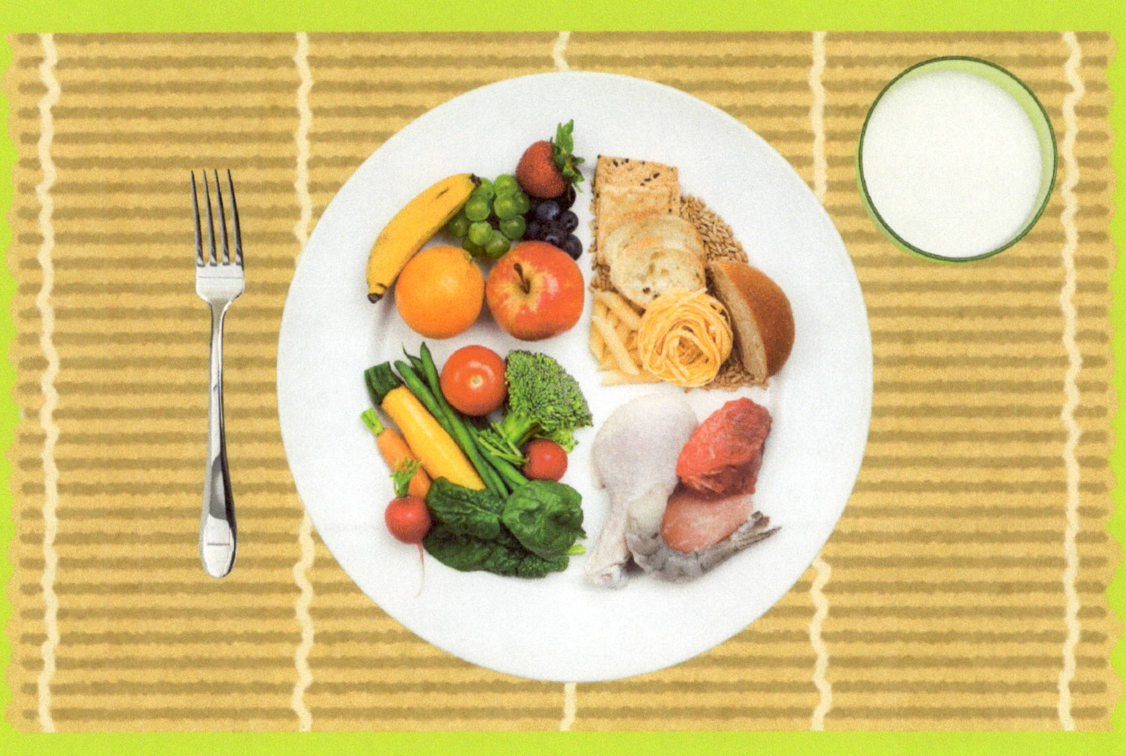

www.ingramcontent.com/pod-product-compliance
Lightning Source LLC
LaVergne TN
LVHW070155110826
845147LV00002B/407

* 9 7 9 8 9 9 3 3 1 4 7 1 6 *